The Care of Children With Long-Term Tracheostomies

The Care of Children With Long-Term Tracheostomies

Ken M. Bleile, Ph.D.

Editor

SINGULAR PUBLISHING GROUP, INC.
San Diego, California

Singular Publishing Group, Inc.
4284 41st Street
San Diego, California 92105-1197

® 1993 by Singular Publishing Group, Inc.

Typeset in 10/12 Palatino by House Graphics
Printed in the United States of America by McNaughton & Gunn

Library of Congress Cataloging-in-Publication Data
The care of children with long-term tracheostomies / Ken M. Bleile, editor.
    p.   cm.
  Includes bibliographical references and index.
  ISBN 1-56593-094-0
  1. Tracheotomy—Patients—Care. 2. Physically handicapped
children—Care.   I. Bleile, Kenneth Mitchell.
  [DNLM: 1. Tracheostomy—in infancy & childhood. 2. Long-Term
Care—infancy & childhood WF 490 C271 1993]
RF517.C35 1993
618.92'097533—dc20
DNLM/DLC
for Library of Congress   93-3951
                                          CIP

CONTENTS

v

CONTRIBUTORS

Elizabeth Barnas, M.S.
Speech-Language Pathologist
Children's Hospital of Buffalo

Ken M. Bleile, Ph.D.*
Assistant Professor
Division of Speech Pathology and
    Audiology
University of Hawaii, Honolulu

Jennifer Buzby-Hadden, M.Ed.
Administrator, Outpatient Services
Children's Seashore House,
    Atlantic City

**Mary Ann Caromano Roberto, B.S.,
    CTRS, CCLS**
Recreational Therapist
Shriners Hospitals for Crippled
    Children,
Philadelphia Unit

Michelle J. Davis, M.S., OTR/L
Occupational Therapist
Private Practice, Philadelphia

Joan Dougherty, RN, BSN
Program Manager, Ventilator Unit
Children's Seashore House,
    Philadelphia

Jean L. Fridy, Ph.D.
Research Associate
Graduate School of Education
    University of Pennsylvania,
    Philadelphia

Laura Fus, M.S.
Predoctoral Fellow
Children's Seashore House,
    Philadelphia

Steven D. Handler, M.D.
Associate Director of Otolaryngology
Children's Hospital of Philadelphia
Associate Professor
Department of Otorhinolaryngology:
    Head and Neck Surgery
University of Pennsylvania School of
    Medicine, Philadelphia

Linda Hock-Long, M.S.S.S., L.S.W.
Program Manager
Child Development Program
Children's Seashore House,
    Philadelphia

Mary Louise Kerwin, Ph.D.
Co-Director, Feeding Team
Children's Seashore House,
    Philadelphia

Deborah Kitley, M.A.
Speech-Language Pathologist
Saint John of God Community
    Services, Philadelphia

Lisa Kurtz, M.Ed., OTR/L
Director of Occupational Therapy
Children's Seashore House,
    Philadelphia

Kathleen Lemanek, Ph.D.
Assistant Professor
Department of Psychology and
    Department of Human
    Development and Family Life
University of Kansas, Lawrence

Stephen Metz, M.D.
Associate Professor
Johns Hopkins School of Medicine,
    Baltimore

---

* formerly Director of Speech-Language Pathology, Children's Seashore House and
  Assistant Professor, Department of Otorhinolaryngology: Head and Neck Surgery,
  University of Pennsylvania School of Medicine

Shari A. Miller, M.A.
Speech-Language Pathologist
Children's Seashore House,
    Philadelphia

John M. Parrish, Ph.D.
Director of Pediatric Psychology
Children's Seashore House,
Philadelphia
Associate Professor
Department of Pediatrics
University of Pennsylvania School of
    Medicine,
Philadelphia

Joy Silverman McGowan, M.S.
Speech-Language Pathologist
Private Practice, Philadelphia

Cynthia Solot, M.A.
Senior Speech-Language Pathologist
Children's Seashore House,
Philadelphia

Meg Stanger, M.S., PT
Director of Program Services
Easter Seal Society of Lancaster
    County,
Pennsylvania

**Symme W. Trachtenberg, M.S.W.,
    L.S.W.**
Director of Social Work
Children's Seashore House,
Philadelphia
Clinical Associate of Social Work in
    Pediatrics
The University of Pennsylvania
    School of Medicine,
Philadelphia

Dolores Vorters, M.S.W., L.S.W.
Social Work Coordinator
Children's Hospital Home Care
    Department
Children's Hospital of Philadelphia

PREFACE

Only two decades ago a child born with a medical condition affecting the airway was likely to die shortly after birth. Today, many of these neonates survive because they are able to breathe through the assistance of long-term tracheostomies. Because of this improvement in medical care, even neonates and infants with severe airway disorders have the opportunity to grow into healthy children and productive adults. However, in most cases this opportunity only becomes a reality after years of medical and developmental interventions.

This book describes the care for children with long-term tracheostomies and is primarily intended for students and professionals in the disciplines most directly involved in the care of these children, including speech-language pathologists, psychologists, occupational therapists, physicians, physical therapists, social workers, nurses, special educators, and recreational therapists. The book contains five sections: Background, Medical Interventions, Developmental Interventions, Care in the Home, and Summary.

Section I is devoted to background on the need for intervention services through a review of the research literature on children with tracheostomies in the areas of morbidity, mortality, developmental outcome, and ethics. The chapters in Section II describe interventions designed to maintain the child's physical health. The author of Chapter 2 discusses medical management of tracheostomy, explaining the reasons for tracheostomy tube placement, the decision-making process involved in preoperative evaluations, surgical techniques, and postoperative care. In Chapter 3 the author describes the medical management of the ventilator.

The chapters in Section III describe developmental interventions designed to improve the quality of life of children with tracheostomies in the areas of motor skills, feeding, communication, behavior, cognition, socialization, and self-help. In Chapter 4 the authors discuss therapies to improve neurodevelopment and motor skills. This chapter also provides a detailed description of the medical precautions required whenever any health care professional provides services to children receiving tracheostomies. The authors of Chapter 5 describe oral-motor and feeding therapies for children with tracheostomies. The authors of Chapter 6 present interventions to facilitate the development of expressive communication in children with tracheostomies with little or no ability to produce speech. Chapter 7 is devoted to interventions for reducing negative psychological ramifications of illness and lengthy hospitalizations on children and their families. Lastly, in Chapter 8 the author describes recreation activities for children with tracheostomies.

The chapters in Section IV address one of the most difficult aspects of care—providing services in the home to children with in-place tracheostomies and ventilators. In Chapter 9 the authors cover the laws establishing the legal basis for providing developmental services. The authors of Chapter 10 describe social services in the hospital and home, along with the organization of care in the home. In Chapter 11 the author describes how to train caregivers to provide physical care to children with in-place tracheostomies. The author of Chapter 12 covers principles to help train a child to self-suction and suggests how these learning principles might be generalized to other care areas.

The book concludes with a summary chapter providing a quick reference guide to major care aspects within this volume. The glossary provides definitions of terminology commonly encountered in the care of children with tracheostomies. In each chapter the first mention of a term defined in the glossary is indicated by **bold face**. The book appendix lists pertinent addresses.

ACKNOWLEDGMENTS

This book is a labor of love, and it is a pleasure to acknowledge the persons who assisted in its development. The authors and editor first must thank the children and their caregivers who inspired this effort. We also thank Singular Publishing Group for agreeing to undertake a book devoted to such a specialized area of care and both the Division of Speech Pathology and Audiology of the University of Hawaii and the Children's Seashore House for providing the resources and encouragement to bring this project to fruition. The editor also extends his thanks to the authors, who undertook their tasks with enthusiasm and a singular lack of concern for turf. More than one author wrote material that he or she then graciously allowed to be placed in another chapter because the switch served the needs of the book. The editor expresses his appreciation to Shari Miller and Laura Fus who served in many ways as editorial assistants and to Marie Linvill of Singular Publishing Group who provided professional and thoughtful guidance of this project from its conception to its completion. The editor also thanks Chiquita Robinson and Yvonne Coleman for providing secretarial assistance far beyond the call of duty. Finally, the editor thanks Terry for making do with a part-time husband for the many months during which this book was written and edited.

SECTION I

BACKGROUND

1

Children With Long-Term Tracheostomies

Ken M. Bleile

INTRODUCTION

This chapter establishes the need for health care services for children with long-term tracheostomies through review of the research literature on mortality, morbidity, developmental outcome, and ethics. The following topics are discussed:

- Estimated prevalence
- Surgical indications
- Mortality rate
- Predictors of developmental outcome
- Intellectual outcome
- Behavioral outcome
- Communication outcome
- Major ethical concerns

CLINICAL CASES

There is a wide range of medical conditions, disabilities, and ethical issues encountered in the provision of care to children with tracheostomies. The two following clinical cases represent composites of several actual children. These cases are used for heuristic purposes throughout this and other chapters to highlight various issues.

Lisa

Lisa was born at 32 weeks, weighing approximately 2,000 g, one of a pair of twin girls. Lisa received **ventilator assistance** at 3 months secondary to **bronchopulmonary dysplasia (BPD)**. While Lisa was in the hospital, she received a variety of therapies, including occupational therapy, speech-language therapy, physical therapy, and recreational therapy. Lisa's nurses provided training to her caregivers in caring for **tracheostomies** in the home, and Lisa's social worker helped the family with adjustment issues.

Lisa was weaned from the ventilator at 9 months and was discharged from the hospital at 11 months. Lisa continued to receive a variety of therapies in the home. After the tracheostomy **cannula** was removed at 14 months, the surgical site remained open, resulting in a weak voice and air leakage. Later, the surgical site was closed and a stronger voice and longer spoken phrases resulted. Lisa's family enrolled her in an early intervention program when she was 2 years old. A psychological evaluation performed at 48 months indicated that Lisa was of normal intelligence (**full-scale IQ** = 94). No behavior problems were observed.

Frank

Frank's mother was an occasional drug abuser when she was pregnant with him. The pregnancy was complicated by first trimester bleeding. Frank was born prematurely at 28 weeks and weighed slightly under 1,500 g. Shortly after birth, Frank was diagnosed as having bronchopulmonary dysplasia, an **intraventricular hemorrhage**, and **gastroesophageal reflux.** Frank received a tracheostomy and ventilator assistance at 3 months.

Frank was transferred from an acute care hospital unit to a rehabilitation unit at 6 months, where, in addition to medical care, he also received services from occupational therapy, physical therapy, speech-language pathology, recreational therapy, psychological help, and social work. At 10 months, Frank was weaned from the ventilator. At 11 months, the child's physician indicated that he was physically able to go home. Frank's family, consisting of his mother and grandmother, had many concerns about having such a "sick child" in their home. The family missed many training sessions on providing home care for Frank. However, training was eventually completed when Frank was 15 months of age, and he was discharged to his home.

During the first months in the home, Frank received 'round the clock nursing care, as well as most of the developmental services he had received in the hospital. The amount of nursing care was gradually reduced over the months as Frank's medical conditions improved and as the family became more comfortable with his care. When Frank's respiratory condition improved, a **laryngotracheoplasty** was performed to treat **subglottic stenosis** and to permit **decannulation.** Finally, at 30 months, Frank's tracheostomy was removed. At 48 months, Frank's full scale intelligence (IQ) was estimated to be 48. Frank's teachers indicated that he had moderate to severe behavior problems.

MEDICAL CHARACTERISTICS

Prevalence

A tracheostomy is an artificial opening between the cervical trachea and the neck. (See Chapter 2.) In this book, a **long-term tracheostomy** is defined as a tracheostomy performed on a child under 13 months of age that is in place for 28 days or longer. A mechanical ventilator is a device that assists or supports the child's lungs in breathing. (See Chapter 3.) The same age and time requirements that are used to define long-term tracheostomy also apply for **long-term (chronic) mechanical ventilation (CMV).**

The Congressional Office of Technology Assessment's 1987 report on children assisted by technology estimates an annual prevalence of 680 to 2,000 children requiring long-term mechanical ventilation (U.S. Congress, 1987). Comparable figures on the prevalence of children receiving long-term tracheostomies are not available. However, one study reports that approximately 70% of its children also received mechanical ventilation (Singer, Kercmar, Legris, Orlowski, Hill, & Doershuk, 1989). If this percentage is representative of that of other centers (an assumption made somewhat questionable given the extensive differences between centers), the number of new patients receiving long-term tracheostomies each year would range from 884 to 2,600.

By definition, the minimum time requirement for a long-term tracheostomy is 1 month. Lisa, the subject of the first case study, had a tracheostomy for 14 months and Frank had a tracheostomy for 30 months. Singer et al. (1989) report that their 130 subjects had tracheostomies in place an average of 15 months (SD = 21 months, range = 1-146 months). The average age at the time of decannulation was 16 months (SD = 20 months, range = 1-144 months). The extreme heterogeneity of the population of children with tracheostomies is indicated by the wide standard deviations within the length of time the children received tracheostomies and, relatedly, the age at which the tracheostomies were removed.

Indications

A variety of medical conditions may give rise to the need for tracheostomy. Further, because of differences between surgeons and hospital populations, a common reason for performing a tracheostomy in one center may be far less common in another location. However, there is a core set of conditions typically cited as rationale for tracheostomy placement (Simon & Silverman McGowan, 1989). These conditions include:

- BPD,
- Subglottic stenosis,
- **Tracheomalacia,**
- **Tracheoesophageal anomaly,**
- **Neuromuscular disorder,**
- **Head trauma,**
- **Congenital anomaly,**
- **Craniofacial anomaly,**
- **Laryngeal neoplasm,**
- **Cardiac anomaly,**
- **Croup,** and
- **Epiglottitis.**

In addition to these conditions, **prematurity** is often associated with tracheostomy placement and the need for ventilator assistance. One recent study reported that half of the children with long-term tracheostomies had been born prematurely (Singer et al., 1989). Additionally, one-third of the total number of subjects in the study had **very low birthweight,** typically defined as less than 1,500 g.

Frank and Lisa both received tracheostomies as a consequence of BPD, a condition often associated with prematurity. BPD and subglottic stenosis are frequently cited indicators of tracheostomy placement (Table 1-1). In four recent studies, BPD is cited as the primary reason for a tracheostomy in 24% to 50% of the total cases. Subglottic stenosis is cited as the indicator in 16% to 47% of the cases (Hill & Singer, 1990; Jennings, 1988; Line, Hawkins, Kahlstrom, McLaughlin, & Ensley, 1986; Simon, Fowler, & Handler, 1983).

TABLE 1-1. Prevalence of BPD and subglottic stenosis (SS) as an indicator for tracheostomy placement.

PERCENTAGE OF CHILDREN	INDICATORS							
	BPD	SS	BPD	SS	BPD	SS	BPD	SS
100								
90								
80								
70								
60								
50								
40						^ ^	+++	^ ^ ^
30			+++			43%	50%	47%
20	+++	^ ^	26%					
10	24%	16%						
0				*	*			

Study: aLine et al. bHill & Singer cJennings dSimon et al.
Year: (1986) (1990) (1988) (1983)
N: .. 25 31 225 77

. = not listed as a diagnostic category
.. = total number of subjects in studies

a From: "Tracheotomy in infants and young children: The changing perspective" by W.S. Line, D. Hawkins, E.J. Kahlstrom, E. McLaughlin, and J. Ensley, 1986, *Laryngoscope, 96*, 510-515.

b From: "Speech and language development after infant tracheostomy" by B. Hill, and L. Singer, (1990), *Journal of Speech and Hearing Disorders, 55*, 15-20.

c From: "Nursing and home aspects of the care of a child with tracheostomy" by P. Jennings, (1988), *Journal of Laryngology and Otology, Supplemental, 17*, 25-29.

d From: "Communication development in young children with long-term tracheostomies: Preliminary report" by B. Simon, S. Fowler, and S. Handler, 1983, *International Journal of Pediatric Otorhinolaryngology, 6*, 37-50.

Reasons for ventilatory assistance are as various as reasons for tracheostomies. A recent study, looking retrospectively at 101 children receiving ventilator assistance, finds that approximately 50% of the children received ventilatory support because of congenital anomalies (Schreiner, Downes, Kettrick, Ise, & Volt, 1987). Of the remaining 50%, approximately 36% had severe BPD and the remaining 15% had neuromuscular disorders.

Mortality Rate

One of the most stressful events for any health care provider is the death of a patient. The mortality rate for children who are tracheostomized and on ventilator assistance falls between 22% to 30% of the total number of patients who receive this surgery (Table 1-2). From 70% to 84% of these deaths occur during the first year after the procedures are performed (Table 1-3). Common causes of

TABLE 1-2. Mortality rates.

PERCENTAGE OF DEATHS	POPULATIONS	
	TRACHEOSTOMY	VENTILATOR ASSISTED
100		
90		
80		
70		
60		
50		
40		
30	++++++++	++++++++
20	++++++++	29% 30%
10	22%	
0		

Study: aLine et al.   bSinger et al.   cSchreiner et al.
Year: (1986)   (1989)   (1987)
N: .   155   130   101
Age of Ss: M = ng ··   5:5   ng
                  S = ng   2:6   ng

· = total number of subjects in studies
·· = information not given (ng)

a From: "Tracheotomy in infants and young children: The changing perspective" by W.S. Line, D. Hawkins, E.J. Kahlstrom, E. McLaughlin, and J. Ensley, 1986, *Laryngoscope, 96*, 510-515.
b From: "Developmental sequelae of long-term infant tracheostomy" by L.T. Singer, C. Kercsmer, G. Legris, J. Orlowski, B. Hill, and C. Doershuk, 1989, *Developmental Medicine and Child Neurology, 31*, 224-230.
c From: "Chronic respiratory failure in infants with prolonged ventilator dependency" by M. Schreiner, J. Downes, R. Kettrick, C. Ise, and R. Volt, 1987, *Journal of the American Medical Association, 258*, 3398-3404.

death include acute lower respiratory infections, worsening underlying conditions, **aspiration, mucus plugging,** and technical failures (Line et al., 1986; Singer et al., 1989). Among patients of Line et al. (1986), approximately 85% of the deaths during the first year after the procedure arose from illness. The remaining 15% arose from complications involving the tracheostomy. In the Schreiner et al. (1987) study of children who were ventilatory assisted, during the first 2 years after the procedure the predominant causes of death were **pulmonary insufficiency** and **cardiac failure.** After the 2-year period, 50% of the deaths resulted from airway and mechanical difficulties with the ventilator.

DEVELOPMENTAL OUTCOME

The feelings of the families of children with long-term tracheostomies evolve over time. When a child first receives a tracheostomy

TABLE 1-3. Percentage of deaths during the first year after surgery.

PERCENTAGE OF DEATHS	POPULATIONS	
	TRACHEOSTOMY	VENTILATOR ASSISTED
100		
90		
80		++++++++ +++++++
70	++++++++ +++++++++	85% 84%
60	70% 70%	
50		
40		
30		
20		
10		
0		

Study:	ₐLine et al.	ᵦSinger et al.	ᵧSchreiner et al.	ᵨFrates et al.

Study: [a]Line et al.   [b]Singer et al.   [c]Schreiner et al.   [d]Frates et al.
Year: (1986)   (1989)   (1987)   (1985)
N: ·   155   130   80 ·   54
Age of
Ss: ·· M = ng ···   5:5   ng   ng
         SD = ng   2:6   ng   ng

·   = survival curve based on first 80 subjects
·· = means and standard deviations are based on total number of subjects
··· = information not given (ng)

[a] From: "Tracheotomy in infants and young children: The changing perspective" by W.S. Line, D. Hawkins, E.J. Kahlstrom, E. McLaughlin, and J. Ensley, 1986, *Laryngoscope, 96*, 510-515.

[b] From: "Developmental sequelae of long-term infant tracheostomy" by L.T. Singer, C. Kercsmer, G. Legris, J. Orlowski, B. Hill, and C. Doershuk, 1989, *Developmental Medicine and Child Neurology, 31*, 224-230.

[c] From: "Chronic respiratory failure in infants with prolonged ventilator dependency" by M. Schreiner, J. Downes, R. Kettrick, C. Ise, and R. Volt, 1987, *Journal of the American Medical Association, 258*, 3398-3404.

[d] From: "Outcome of home mechanical ventilation in children" R.C. Frates, M.L. Spaingard, E.O. Smith, and G.M. Harrison, 1985, *The Journal of Pediatrics, 106*, 850-856.

or ventilator assistance, caregivers and family are often happy just that the child is alive. Later, caregivers naturally begin to wonder about their child's future. Seeing their child lying in a crib, breathing through a new opening in the neck, caregivers often report feeling haunted by such questions as: Will my child lead a normal life? What about retardation? Will my baby ever talk? And if my child lacks the ability to self-care, what happens to my youngster when I am gone?

In many circumstances, children who receive long-term tracheostomies have a good prognosis for future development. In such cases, information on developmental outcome can relieve anxiety and help caregivers begin to look past a difficult present into a better future. When the prognosis appears to be less than good, information on long-term outcome may begin to help caregivers make the first step toward acceptance and accommodation. In conveying information on developmental outcome to caregivers, it should be remembered that outcome data on a population do not define an individual child's potential. Every experienced clinician can cite many cases in which a child defied the odds and ended up much better than expected. Alternately, every clinician can report cases where the prognostic indicators were good, but the child's developmental outcome was poor.

Predictors

There are several readily identifiable predictors of future developmental outcome for children with tracheostomies and those receiving ventilator assistance. First, the longer the tracheostomy is in place, the poorer a child's eventual developmental outcome is likely to be. This is because children with more severe illnesses are likely to have the tracheostomy in place for longer periods of time. Further, longer placement offers more opportunities for episodes of **anoxia.** Second, the lower the birthweight the more likely it is that the child will experience later developmental problems. This is because low birth weight children are more likely to experience **neurological sequelae** than are children in the general population. In babies born with birthweights of less than 1,500 g, 13% to 30% of the surviving infants have intellectual abilities that fall within the range of mental retardation (Bernbaum & Hoffman-Williamson, 1991).

Intelligence

One of the most difficult questions asked by caregivers is: Will my child be retarded? The authors of a recent study of the developmental outcome of children with tracheostomies found that approximately half (49%) the children had normal intelligence (Singer et al., 1989). The average IQ of these children was 92.1, and the standard deviation (average distance from the mean) was 14.5. Among the general population, the average IQ is 100 and the standard deviation is 15. A combination of reasons probably determine the IQ difference of even children with tracheostomies of normal intelligence from the general population. Likely explanations include the existence of medical conditions precipitating the tracheostomy, and ongoing illnesses and episodes of anoxia while the tracheostomy was in place.

The remaining 51% of the Singer et al. subjects (1989) were mentally retarded (Table 1-4). Six percent of these children were mildly retarded and the intelligence of the remaining 45% of the children ranged from moderately to profoundly retarded. The most common conditions associated with mental retardation among children with tracheostomies were prematurity, seizures, **asphyxia,** and very low birthweight (Table 1-5). Other conditions associated with mental retardation included **Down syndrome, quadriplegia, myelomeningocele,** and **hydrocephalus** (Singer et al., 1989).

Schreiner et al. (1987) assessed the developmental outcomes of children receiving ventilator assistance (Table 1-6). The children's developmental outcomes were divided into five categories: normal, borderline, mild delay, moderate delay, and severe delay. Approximately 48% of the children were found to have normal or borderline development. The development of the other approximately 52% ranged from mildly to severely delayed.

Lastly, Gunn, Lepore, and Outerbridge (1983) studied the developmental outcome of 103 children assisted by ventilators. The

TABLE 1-4. Intellectual outcome in surviving children with tracheostomies.

PERCENTAGE OF DEATHS	INTELLIGENCE		
	AVERAGE RANGE	MILDLY RETARDED	MODERATELY TO PROFOUNDLY RETARDED
100			
90			
80			
70			
60			
50	++++++++		
40	49%		++++++++
30			45%
20			
10		++++++++	
0		6%	

Study: aSinger et al.
Year: (1989)
N: 65 .
Age of Ss: .. M = 5:5
                  SD = 2:6

. = number of children with long-term tracheostomies who survived and were not lost to follow up

.. = means and standard deviations are based on total number of subjects

a From: "Developmental sequelae of long-term infant tracheostomy" by L.T. Singer, C. Kercsmer, G. Legris, J. Orlowski, B. Hill, and C. Doershuk, 1989, *Developmental Medicine and Child Neurology, 31,* 224-230.

TABLE 1-5. Medical diagnoses of long-term tracheostomy survivors with mental retardation.

DIAGNOSIS	NUMBER	PERCENTAGE
Preterm, seizures, asphyxia, very low birthweight	10	34%
Down syndrome	4	14%
Quadriplegia	4	14%
Myelomeningocele and hydrocephalus	2	7%
Other	9	31%

Study: aSinger et al.
Year: (1989)
N: 29 .
Age of Ss: .. M = 5:5
           SD = 2:6

· = number of children with mental retardation
.. = means and standard deviations are based on total number of subs.

a From: "Developmental sequelae of long-term infant tracheostomy" by L.T. Singer, C. Kercsmer, G. Legris, J. Orlowski, B. Hill, and C. Doershuk, 1989, *Developmental Medicine and Child Neurology, 31*, 224-230.

TABLE 1-6. Developmental outcomes of surviving children who received ventilator assistance.

PERCENTAGE OF CHILDREN	DEVELOPMENTAL OUTCOME				
	NORMAL	BORDER-LINE	MILD DELAY	MODERATE DELAY	SEVERE DELAY
100					
90					
80					
70					
60					
50					
40					
30	+++				
20	32%	+++	+++	+++	+++
10		16%	18%	18%	16%
0				*	*

Study: aSchreiner et al.
Year: (1987)
N: 56.
Age of Ss: .. M = ng ...
           SD = ng

· = number of surviving patients whose developmental outcome could be assessed
.. =. means and standard deviations are based on total number of subjects
... = information not given (ng)

a From: "Chronic respiratory failure in infants with prolonged ventilator dependency" by M. Schreiner, J. Downes, R. Kettrick, C. Ise, and R. Volt, 1987, *Journal of the American Medical Association, 258*, 3398-3404.

patients were aged between 5 and 12 at the time of follow-up. Psychometric assessment indicated that (84%) of the children had approximately normal distribution of intelligence relative to the general population. Four percent of the children were found to have minor neurological handicaps, and 7% had sufficient neurological handicaps to preclude school attendance. Poorer neurological sequelae were found to be associated significantly with **perinatal** asphyxia and birthweights of 1,500 g or less.

Behavior

Behavior problems are not uncommon among children who have undergone long-term tracheostomies. Approximately 50% of children with tracheostomies with normal intelligence demonstrate either behavior problems or social isolation (Singer et al., 1989). We can only conjecture that these children's often rocky medical courses seem likely to contribute to such difficulties. Further, these children are often reared under extraordinary circumstances, including lengthy hospitalizations, and, even after returning to the community, frequent hospital readmissions for varying lengths of time. When home, medical problems may make bonding between the child and family difficult and may inhibit normal social experiences with other children. Under these conditions, it is surprising that more children do not have behavior problems.

At present no data exist on the prevalence of behavior problems among children with tracheostomies who also are mentally retarded. Behavior problems are relatively frequent among children with mental retardation. The exceptional medical and social circumstances of these children may lead one to hypothesize that these children might have more behavior problems than other children with mental retardation. However, more research is needed before we know with certainty that such is the case.

Communication

One of the most direct results of a tracheostomy is interference in communication development. While the tracheostomy is in place, children often have limited ability to communicate. The limitation is due in large measure to the tracheostomy itself, which can make vocalization difficult or impossible. Additionally, the combination of the child's illness, social setting, and tracheostomy can severely interfere with the child's ability to learn the language skills necessary to express ideas and feelings.

Nonetheless, the long-term prognosis for speech and language development appears good (Table 1-7). At approximately 5 years old, the language development of virtually all children who previously received tracheostomies or ventilator assistance is commensurate with their **nonverbal intelligence.** Additionally, approximately 83% to 87% of these children have speech abilities on a par with their level of language development.

In considering the relatively optimistic outcome data for the development of communication, the following issues should be kept in mind. First, virtually all the children studied received extensive intervention services for their communication difficulties. Most investigators would likely conclude that such interventions are necessary to achieve outcomes as good as found in the children. Second, the studies do not compare these children to youngsters their own age. Rather, the studies compare each child's speech and

TABLE 1-7. Percentage of children receiving tracheostomies with normal speech and language development.

PERCENTAGE OF CHILDREN	POPULATIONS			
	Normal Intelligence		Both Normal and Retarded Children	
	SPEECH	LANGUAGE	SPEECH	LANGUAGE
100		+++++		+++++
90		100%	+++++	100%
80	+++++		87%	
70	83%			
60				
50				
40				
30				
20				
10				
0				

Study: [a]Hill and Singer   [b]Simon, Fowler, and Handler
Year: 1990   1983
N: 23 (speech) ·   23 (speech and language) ··
            31 (language) ···
Age of Ss: ···· M = 5.3   ng ·····
                 SD = 2.3   ng

· = number of testable surviving children
·· = number of children for whom follow up data were available
··· = total number of subjects in study
···· = means and standard deviations are based on total number of subjects
····· = information not given (ng)

[a] From: "Speech and language development after infant tracheostomy" by B. Hill and L. Singer, (1990), *Journal of Speech and Hearing Disorders, 55,* 15-20.
[b] From: "Communication development in young children with long-term tracheostomies: Preliminary report" by B. Simon, S. Fowler, and S. Handler, 1983, *International Journal of Pediatric Otorhinolaryngology, 6,* 37-50.

language development to the youngster's own nonverbal abilities. Actually, many of these children appear delayed relative to children their own age. Lastly, Hill and Singer (1990) note that their subjects may have had language delays on entering school. However, as the authors observe, the performance disparity may have resulted from the fact that different evaluation instruments were employed to test the school-age children and the younger children. Future research is needed to determine whether children who previously received tracheostomies experience language and learning disabilities as academic demands increase during the school years.

ETHICAL CONCERNS

The care of children with long-term tracheostomies gives rise to a number of perplexing ethical concerns. Indeed, the situation of children with long-term tracheostomies, although a new clinical population, poses some very old and troubling ethical questions. These questions include who should decide when a person lives or dies, and what obligations does a society have to provide care to its less fortunate members. How these questions are answered in no small way defines a culture and a person. Refusal to address ethical issues is, itself, a type of defining answer.

Issues of life and death are most likely to arise in acute care hospital settings as the extent of a child's medical difficulties becomes clear. In the case of children such as Frank, who have neurologic components to their disability, the underlying condition is usually irreversible and often progressive. However, the condition may not be a threat to life. Whether a child who is very ill with an illness that is not life threatening should be "allowed" to die is one of the most complex ethical questions in our time.

Although life and death issues can arise at any point in the care of children with tracheostomies, ethical issues in rehabilitation hospitals and in community educational settings are more likely to involve provision of therapy services. Although either Frank or Lisa could serve to illustrate these issues, a better example is H, a child with profound mental retardation.

H

H was a full-term child born with severe respiratory, physical, and cognitive deficits. H has been ventilated since birth and now, at age 5, has always lived in a small community hospital. H eats three pureed meals a day. The youngster can walk independently with a somewhat awkward gait. H's fine motor abilities are limited by a significantly smaller left hand. H communicates through signing. However, the signs are "sloppy" and generally are only understood in context by those who know the child. H's behavior problems include self-abuse and aggression toward others. Recently, a bed in a state hospital became available. The state hospital is well staffed with doctors and nurses and would be a safe physical environment for H. However, everyone acknowledges that the developmental therapies offered in the state hospital are poor, and that H's development would likely languish if transferred there. H's caregivers have legal custody, but have not seen H in 3 years. The caregivers have indicated that they will follow whatever course the hospital recommends.

Based on the information above, it is relatively clear that the community hospital has the legal right to transfer H to the state hospital. The ethical question is whether the community hospital is justified in sending H to a setting where the youngster's development is likely to be affected adversely. An argument in favor of the transfer is that H's departure would open the bed in the community hospital for another child. Thus, keeping H in the community hospital, in effect, denies services to some other child. Additionally, the state hospital is a safe environment, even though it is regrettable that it does not provide the best environment for development. A counterargument to transferring H might be that the community hospital has a greater ethical obligation to care for H than for other children. This is because the community hospital, though not H's legal guardian, has assumed a parental role through its long association with H. Because the hospital is filling a parental role, it has an ethical obligation to look after H's best interest.

Although the above illustration describes a situation in a hospital, the principles involved are equally applicable in an educational setting. In effect, the question such children as H pose is what obligation does society have to help the children its technology has saved?

In the vast majority of cases, the ethical issues arising during the care of children with tracheostomies are resolved by the child's care-givers or legal guardians. Depending on the issues involved, other participants may include the child's physician, the family's minister or rabbi, a social worker, a family friend, or an educator. However, at times caregivers or health care providers may seek more formal assistance. Such cases may be presented to an ethics committee.

A recent study from a major children's hospital found that approximately 50% of the cases sent to its ethics committee involved the use of mechanical ventilation (Michaels & Oliver, 1986). In such cases the purpose of the ethics committee is to provide the child's caregivers and health care providers an objective and thoughtful viewpoint. The committees hearing these cases typically comprise caregivers of children with disabilities, religious persons, community members, and members of the health care system.

Ethics committees might approach the types of cases described above from any number of perspectives. In considering whether caregivers should "allow" their child to die, an ethics committee would be likely to focus on making certain that the child's caregivers have been informed regarding the child's prognosis for future health and development. The ethics committee would also likely want to be certain that the caregivers have an opportunity to deliberate on these matters in as calm and supportive environment as possible.

In considering such cases as H, an ethics committee would likely observe that H, lacking an advocate whose function is to look after her best interests, is at a disadvantage. The community hospital cannot play such a role because a conflict exists between its desire to care for H and its mission to provide bed space to care for other children. A possible recommendation of an ethics committee would be to appoint an advocate for H and other children requiring long-term care in the hospital. The advocate, who might be a member of the clergy, would serve the function of acting in H's behalf.

CONCLUSIONS

The motivation to provide health care services to children with tracheostomies is based on the existence of disabilities among these children. Many children who have been tracheostomized have severe neurological and physical deficits, and the tracheostomy and ventilator themselves, may, although providing life-saving services, also contribute to disability. The physical and developmental problems of these children range from mild to severe.

Providing health care services to children with tracheostomies raises both ethical and organizational challenges. The ethical dilemmas begin with life and death concerns in the neonatal intensive care unit and evolve into provision of care issues in the rehabilitation hospital and community. The organization of health care services is dictated by the complex nature of these children's medical issues and developmental problems, requiring a team approach in order to provide all necessary areas of care. Review of the research literature indicates that a health care team providing services to children with tracheostomies must be prepared to address disabilities in such diverse realms as physical care, motor skills, communication, behavior, movement, cognition, and socialization.

REFERENCES

Bernbaum, J., & Hoffman-Williamson, M. (1991). *Primary care of the preterm infant.* St. Louis: Mosby Year Book.

Fowler, S., Simon, B., & Handler, S. (1983). Communication development in young children with long-term tracheostomies: A preliminary report. *International Journal of Otorhinolaryngology, 6,* 37-50.

Frates, R.C., Spaingard, M.L., Smith, E.O., & Harrison, G.M. (1985). Outcome of home mechanical ventilation in children. *The Journal of Pediatrics, 106,* 850-856.

Gunn, T., Lepore, E., & Outerbridge, E. (1983). Outcome at school age after neonatal mechanical ventilation. *Developmental Medicine and Child Neurology, 25,* 305-314.

Hill, B., & Singer, L. (1990). Speech and language development after infant tracheostomy. *Journal of Speech and Hearing Disorders, 55,* 15-20.

Jennings, P. (1988). Nursing and home aspects of the care of a child with tracheostomy. *Journal of Laryngology and Otology,* (Suppl. 17), 25-29.

Line, W.S., Hawkins, D., Kahlstrom, E.J., McLaughlin, E., & Ensley, J. (1986). Tracheotomy in infants and young children: The changing perspective. *Laryngoscope, 96,* 510-515.

Locke, J. (1983). *Phonological acquisition and change.* New York: Academic Press.

Locke, J., & Pearson, D. (1990). Linguistic significance of babbling: Evidence from a tracheostomized infant. *Journal of Child Language, 17,* 1-16.

Michaels, R.H., & Oliver, T.K. (1986). Human rights consultation: A twelve-year experience of a pediatric bioethics committee. *Pediatrics, 78,* 566-572.

Oller, K., & Eilers, R. (1988). The role of audition in infant babbling. *Child Development, 59,* 441-449.

Saletsky Kamen, R., & Watson, B. (1991). Effects of long-term tracheostomy on spectral characteristics of vowel production. *Journal of Speech and Hearing Research, 34,* 1057-1065.

Schreiner, M., Downes, J., Kettrick, R., Ise, C., & Volt, R. (1987). Chronic respiratory failure in infants with prolonged ventilator dependency. *Journal of the American Medical Association, 258,* 3398-3404.

Simon, B., Fowler, S., & Handler, S. (1983). Communication development in young children with long-term tracheostomies: Preliminary report. *International Journal of Pediatric Otorhinolaryngology, 6,* 37-50.

Simon, B., & Silverman McGowan, J. (1989). Tracheotomy in young children: Implications for assessment and treatment of communication and feeding disorders. *Infants and Young Children, 1,* 1-9.

Singer, L.T., Kercsmer, C., Legris, G., Orlowski, J., Hill, B., & Doershuk, C. (1989). Developmental sequelae of long-term infant tracheostomy. *Developmental Medicine and Child Neurology, 31,* 224-230.

Stark, R. (1980). Stages of speech development in the first year of life. In G. Yeni-Komshian, J. Kavanagh, & C. Ferguson (Eds.), *Child phonology: Production*. New York: Academic Press.

U.S. Congress, Office of Technology Assessment. (1987, May). Technology-dependent children: Hospital v. home care—a technical memorandum. OTA-TM-H-38, U.S. Government Printing Office.

SECTION II

MEDICAL INTERVENTIONS

2

Surgical Management of the Tracheostomy

Steven D. Handler

INTRODUCTION

In this chapter, the surgical management of the tracheostomy is described. The following topics are discussed:

• Medical conditions that require a tracheostomy
• The effects of the tracheostomy tube on vocalization
• Important aspects of the surgical procedure
• Aspects of postoperative care and management

REASONS FOR TRACHEOSTOMY

A tracheostomy is an artificial opening created between the trachea and the neck (Figure 2-1). A **cannula** of metal or plastic is inserted through the anterior neck and into the **tracheal lumen** below the larynx (and, thus, below the vocal folds). The child inspires air through the tracheostomy tube (voluntarily or by means of **mechanical ventilation**) and into the lungs. If the tracheostomy cannula fits tightly in the tracheal lumen, all of the child's air is exhaled out through the tracheostomy tube. There is no ability to phonate, because no air passes up through the vocal cords. If there is sufficient room in the tracheal lumen between the tracheostomy tube and the tracheal wall, air can be exhaled up around the cannula and through the vocal cords. This permits vocalization to occur on exhalation.

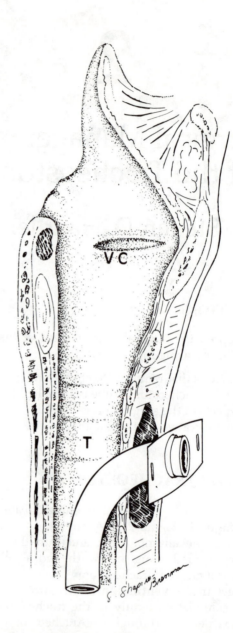

Figure 2-1. Tracheostomy tube in place in cervical trachea (T). Note relationship below vocal cords (VC). From "The speech pathologist and management of children with tracheostomies" by B. Simon and S. Handler, 1981, *Journal of Otolaryngology, 10,* 440-448. Copyright 1981 by S. Handler. Reprinted by permission.

There are three primary indications for tracheostomy: (1) **long-term mechanical ventilation,** (2) to bypass airway obstruction, and (3) to facilitate **tracheobronchial toilet** (Wetmore, Handler, & Potsic, 1982). The child requiring a **long-term tracheostomy** may have any one or a combination of the three reasons for the procedure. The vast majority of children that require long-term tracheostomies have respiratory distress syndrome secondary to **bronchopulmonary dysplasia (BPD)** (such as, for example, Lisa and Frank, see Chapter 1). These children will require long-term ventilation from weeks and months to years. Although an **endotracheal tube** can serve this purpose for a short time, the risk of developing **subglottic stenosis** increases significantly after **endotracheal intubation** of several weeks. Consequently, neonates requiring ventilation for longer than 6-8 weeks should have tracheostomies performed to continue the ventilatory assistance and to minimize development of subglottic stenosis. The length of time a child can tolerate intubation decreases with growth so that a child older than 1 year would be allowed to be intubated for only 2-3 weeks before a tracheostomy was considered. This difference in susceptibility to subglottic stenosis is thought to be that infants tolerate intubation for a longer period of time without suffering any damage and because of soft, yielding neonate laryngeal tissue.

Airway obstruction, the second indication for tracheostomy, can be congenital or acquired. A small percentage of children are born with congenital laryngeal anomalies, such as subglottic stenosis, **webs,** vocal cord paralysis, or **laryngomalacia.** Children with cranio-facial anomalies such as **Pierre Robin syndrome** or **Treacher Collins' syndrome** also fall into this category. In these children, the lower airway or lungs may be adequately developed, but the upper airway is insufficient to allow passage of air. Acquired lesions such as subglottic stenosis are, unfortunately, not that uncommon after long-term endotracheal intubation and result in the need for long-term tracheostomy even though the child has outgrown the BPD.

The third category of patients requiring long-term tracheostomy is children with **neuromuscular disorders** unable to handle their own respiratory secretions. These children need a constant tracheobronchial toilet that can be delivered for only a few weeks through the endotracheal tube. Long-term management of airway secretions requires a tracheostomy. The tube permits easy access to the lower airway to **aspirate** secretions. The reason for a tracheostomy may change as a child progresses through the course of medical care. For example, a child who requires tracheostomy for long-term ventilation may still require the tracheostomy to bypass subglottic stenosis even when ventilatory support requirement has decreased. The dynamic nature of the child's respiratory status and consequent airway requirements cannot be overemphasized. As a patient's condition changes, the requirements for the size of the tracheostomy tube change, the need for use of mechanical ventilation may vary, and the opportunity to use a **fenestrated cannula** or a **speaking valve** may present itself.

TRACHEOSTOMY TUBES

The choice of tracheostomy tube is largely a matter of surgeon preference (Figure 2-2). Some surgical specialists still use the double lumen metal tubes in use since the 1930s. The system allows for removal of the inner cannula for cleaning while maintaining the airway with the outer cannula. However, the newer plastic materials have minimized the incidence of plugging and are less traumatic to the soft tracheal tissues of children. Therefore, most otolaryngologists use tubes of commercially available silastic or Polyvinylchloride (PVC).

Each child must be considered individually when a tracheostomy is planned. The proposed length of time that the tracheostomy tube is to be in place, the need for ventilation, the need for tracheobronchial toilet, and other associated medical questions all need to be considered in preoperatively evaluating the child. Although there are guidelines matching the size of tracheostomy tube with ages of children, the actual requirements of each child can vary depending on physical condition (age and size) and respiratory requirements. A child requiring high ventilatory pressures or constant tracheobronchial suctioning will need as large a tube as possible to facilitate these functions. Another child who has only subglottic stenosis may not require such a large tube. Actually, a slightly smaller tube would be preferable in the latter case, as it would allow for air passage alongside the cannula to permit vocalization.

The sizes of the old style metal and some of the plastic tracheostomy tubes are listed by Jackson size (#000, 00, 0, 1, 2, etc.). However, the Jackson sizes are not readily transferable to millimeter equivalents, and it is not easy to use this nomenclature to determine the appropriate size tube for a specific infant or child. The more modern plastic tubes are all labeled with millimeter sizes, usually internal and external diameter.

In some of the brands of tracheostomy tubes, there are neonatal and infant lengths available, so even the smallest child can have a

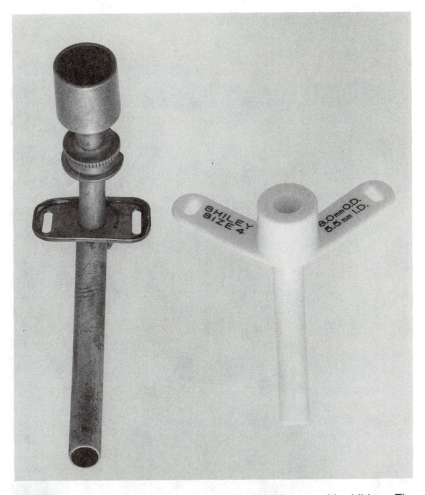

Figure 2-2. Two of the tracheostomy tubes now in use with children. The metal tube on the left has an inner cannula that fits inside the outer tube.

tube of appropriate length. The tips of the tracheostomy tube should lie approximately 1 cm above the **carina** trachea. However, in some styles, neonatal lengths are not available and the tracheostomy tube must be custom cut to fit the individual child. It is important that all members of the health care team know if a tube has been modified, so that a replacement tube can be cut to the same specifications.

If the reason for the tracheostomy is long-term ventilation, a special adapter to connect the tracheostomy tube to the ventilator must be employed. Several adapter styles are available having multiple points of articulation to allow the child to move freely without torquing the tracheostomy tube (Figure 2-3). This is

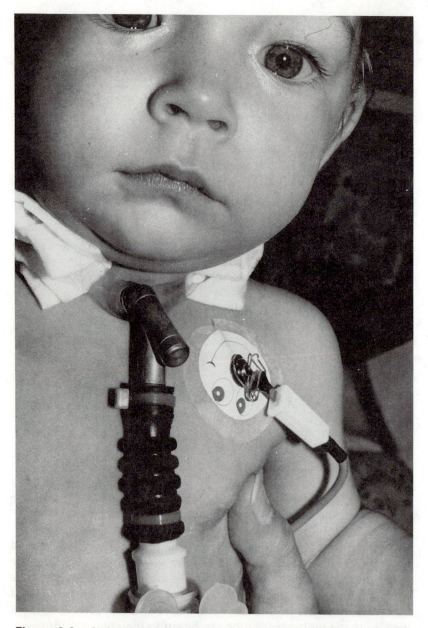

Figure 2-3. Articulated connector between tracheostomy tube and anesthesia circuit allows greater freedom of movement.

especially important for infants who like to be prone and need to develop upper body strength and coordination through crawling.

PROCEDURE

When the decision is made to perform a long-term tracheos-tomy, the operation is rarely performed on an emergency basis. The surgical specialist performing the tracheostomy can be an otolaryn-gologist, general surgeon, or thoracic surgeon, depending on experience and expertise with airway problems in children. In the operating room, adequate preparation should be made to perform this procedure with the necessary personnel present to assist. Although the procedure can be performed in an ICU, the wide, nonadjusting ICU bed and the absence of all the equipment and supplies usually present in an operating room make this a less than ideal site.

The procedure is performed with the patient intubated or ventilated through a rigid **bronchoscope** (Figure 2-4A). The patient is placed supine on the operating room table with a roll placed under the shoulders to extend the head and neck. This brings the cervical trachea up against the anterior neck skin. A horizontal skin incision is used because of its superior cosmetic result. Stay sutures of silk are placed lateral to the proposed tracheostomy incision to aid in replacement of the tube in the event of accidental decannu-lation postoperatively (Figure 2-4B). A vertical incision is made in the trachea through the second, third, and fourth tracheal rings, with the tracheostomy tube placed in the trachea as the endotra-cheal tube or bronchoscope is withdrawn (Figure 2-4C).

The tracheostomy tube is secured with cotton (or cotton Velcro) ties around the neck (Figure 2-4D). Foam padding is used to protect the neck skin from abrasion secondary to the ties. The tracheostomy tube is not sutured in place because that might make recannulation much more difficult following the event of accidental **decannulation.**

POSTOPERATIVE CARE

Postoperative tracheostomy care is very critical for the first 7 days after surgery. A chest radiograph is obtained to detect any possible **pneumothorax** and to document tracheostomy tube position in relation to the carina. Also, postoperative care for the first week is directed to keeping the tracheostomy tube open and patent to minimize risk of accidental decannulation, a disastrous occurrence during this period. Within this first postoperative week, the **tracheostomy tube tract** (connection between neck skin and tracheal lumen through which the tracheostomy tube passes) is not well formed and accidental decannulation would cause soft tissue to

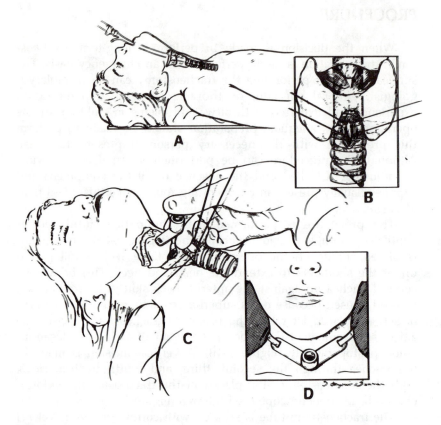

Figure 2-4. (A) Patient in supine position for tracheostomy. The neck is extended on a shoulder roll. Note position of skin incision (dotted line). (B) Vertical incision in trachea. Note lateral stay sutures to be used in the event of accidental decannulation. (C) Tracheostomy tube is inserted into trachea. (D) Tracheostomy tube secured with neck ties.

immediately close over the operative site. Therefore, any manipulation of the freshly placed tracheostomy tube must be kept to a minimum. If speech-language consultation is obtained for these patients, the therapist is asked to make the initial evaluation after the first tracheostomy tube change which is usually performed 1 week postoperatively. By this time, the tracheostomy tract is usually well formed and accidental decannulation should not pose such a significant problem. However, any health care professional involved with a child with a tracheostomy must be aware that manipulation of the tube by the therapist or even by the child may result in accidental decannulation. The health care professional must be aware of the signs of accidental decannulation—(**cyanosis, air**

hunger, significant change in heart rate, vocalization around a tracheostomy tube in a child who has been aphonic)—and how to summon help in such an event.

When replacing a tracheostomy tube, it is important for the caregivers to know the correct position that the child must be in to facilitate replacement of the tube. The child is placed on a rolled towel or sheet with the head extended on the neck. This brings the neck skin and trachea to the same orientation created during the original surgical procedure. This straightens the tracheostomy tract and allows for easy replacement of the tracheostomy cannula.

Routine tracheostomy tube changes after the initial change are performed at regular intervals determined by the individual patient. Although some institutions recommend weekly and even daily tracheostomy tube changes, we believe that for children without significant problems of thick secretions and/or plugging, the tube may be changed every 2-3 weeks. Of course, this regimen should not be rigid and should be adapted to changes in the child's condition and for any associated upper respiratory infection. It is important that the various caregivers know how to change or replace a tracheostomy tube should it become plugged or accidentally displaced.

As the child grows and the youngster's medical condition improves, the requirements for the tracheostomy tube may change. If the child once needed a tight-fitting tracheostomy tube to permit high pressure ventilation, improved pulmonary condition may allow for a looser fitting tube, permitting vocalization. In addition, as the youngster grows, a modified (cut) tube may be replaced by a full-length standard tube.

Meticulous attention must be paid to the **stoma,** the area around the cannula, to be kept clean and dry. If this site breaks down, it can be a source of constant infection and pain for the child. This can affect both feeding and voice production. Granulation tissue may form around this stoma from inflammation around the foreign body (tracheostomy cannula). Although this usually can be minimized by use of topical steroid-antibiotic ointments, occasionally silver nitrate must be used to treat this granulation tissue. If the granulation becomes large, it can block the stoma when the tracheostomy cannula is withdrawn and can impede replacement of the tube (Figure 2-5). If this happens, the granuloma must be surgically excised. Rarely, **hypertrophic scarring** around the stoma can create a **keloid**-type lesion. If the keloid prevents access to the stoma, this, too, must be surgically removed.

Occasionally, a small amount of granulation tissue may form inside the trachea just superior to the tracheostomy tube (Handler,

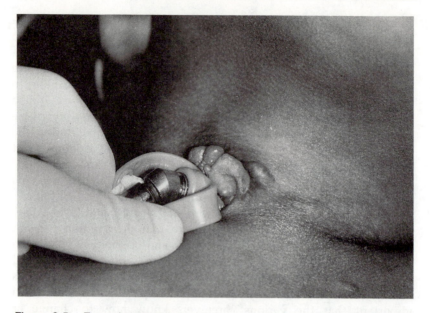

Figure 2-5. Extensive granulation tissue surrounding tracheostomy stoma.

1986). This usually causes no problem. However, if this granuloma enlarges, it can completely fill the tracheal lumen and obstruct the upper airway (Figure 2-6). Although this is not of importance when the tracheostomy tube is in place, it can contribute to severe airway distress, if the tracheostomy tube becomes obstructed or displaced, by preventing respiration through the larynx. In addition, blockage of the upper airway can reduce or eliminate vocalization in a manner similar to severe subglottic stenosis complication. Therefore, endoscopic evaluation of the upper airway is recommended at approximately 6-month intervals to assess laryngeal function, the subglottic space, and the presence of any granulation tissue or obstructing lesion that could affect voice and/or respiration. Intratracheal granulomas are removed surgically during these procedures.

VOCALIZATION WITH THE TRACHEOSTOMY TUBE

Although some children can vocalize around the tracheostomy tube, many are unable to vocalize with a tracheostomy tube in place (Simon & Handler, 1981). The most common cause for inability to vocalize is subglottic stenosis from long-term intubation that preceded the tracheostomy (Figure 2-7). Another determinate is a

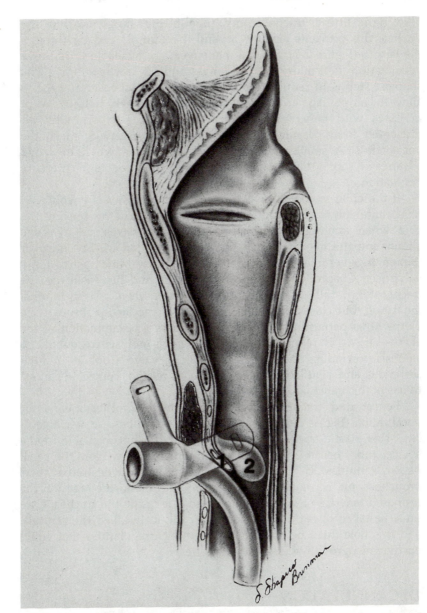

Figure 2-6. Small amount of granulation tissue (1) at superior edge of stoma. Large granuloma (2), completely obstructing tracheal lumen. From "Difficult decannulation" by S. Handler, 1986. In G. Gates (Ed.), *Current therapy in otolaryngology—Head and neck surgery* (pp. 327-329). Philadelphia: B.C. Decker. Copyright 1986 by S. Handler. Reprinted by permission.

very tight fitting tracheostomy tube fitting snugly within the trachea; this prevents air flow around the cannula and up through the larynx (Figure 2-7). Several maneuvers are available to improve vocalization in children with long-standing tracheostomy. The simplest step is to reduce the diameter of the tracheostomy tube to allow for air passage around the cannula. This is very helpful except in cases with concomitant severe subglottic stenosis, with air prevented from passing through the narrow airway to reach the vocal cords. A smaller cannula is not acceptable when the child requires a large diameter tracheostomy tube for high pressure ventilation.

If the child is cooperative enough, the youngster is encouraged to occlude the tracheostomy tube with a finger or by tucking the chin when attempting to vocalize. Speaking valves are available eliminating the need for such patient cooperation in the endeavor (Simon & Silverman McGowan, 1989). The Passy-Muir tracheostomy valve (see Chapter 6) is such an apparatus and fits easily on the tracheostomy tube. The diaphragm on the valve allows normal inhalation, but closes on exhalation to force the air up through the glottis, thus permitting vocalization. Endoscopic examination of the child's airway is required to assure there is not severe subglottic stenosis precluding use of such a speaking valve. Copious tracheal secretions and ventilator requirements are relative contraindications to use of this valve.

Fenestrated tracheostomy tubes provide another means for vocalization (Figure 2-8). Although fenestrated tubes are available in large-size plastic tracheostomy tubes, they are not available in the smaller tubes because the fenestra can structurally weaken the small plastic cannulas. If it is decided to employ a fenestrated tube, bronchoscopy is required to identify and mark the site of the proposed fenestra on the cannula when it is inside the trachea. Care must be taken to cut a small hole that will not weaken the cannula, and this hole must be smooth and without irregularities that could encourage ingrowth of granulation tissue.

DECANNULATION

Readiness for decannulation must be determined medically and with an endoscopic examination. If the child's mechanical ventilation requirements have ceased, endoscopic examination of the upper airway must be performed before decannulation to assess laryngeal function, adequacy of the subglottic space, and absence of any intratracheal pathology that could cause respiratory obstruction.

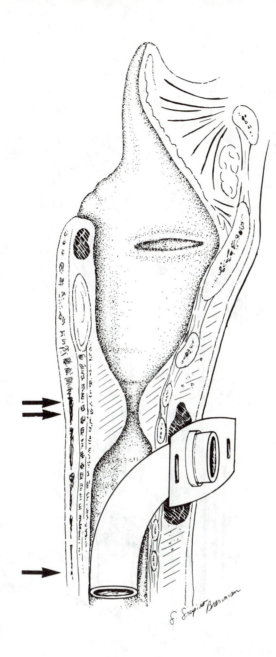

Figure 2-7. Tight-fitting tracheostomy tube (single arrow) or subglottic stenosis (double arrows) can impede flow of air past vocal cords and prevent vocalization. From "The speech pathologist and management of children with tracheostomies" by B. Simon and S. Handler, 1981, *Journal of Otolaryngology, 10,* 440-448. Copyright 1981 by S. Handler. Reprinted with permission.

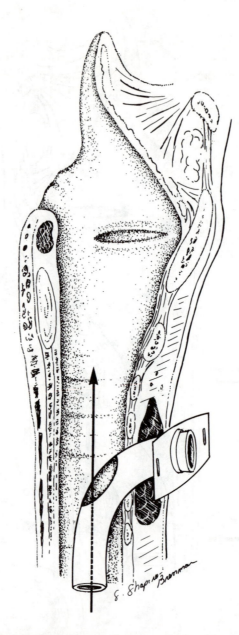

Figure 2-8. Fenestrated tracheostomy tube permits flow of air up through tube past the vocal cords to permit vocalization. From "The speech pathologist and management of children with tracheostomies" by B. Simon and S. Handler, 1981, *Journal of Otolaryngology, 10,* 440-448. Copyright 1981 by S. Handler. Reprinted with permission.

Severe subglottic stenosis will prevent successful decannulation, but mild stenosis (less than 30% restriction of tracheal airway) may improve with time or after periodic endoscopic dilatations (stretching). Formal repair of the stenosis has the greatest degree of success. **Laryngotracheoplasty** (Figure 2-9) is a procedure in which the narrowed and scarred airway is surgically opened and a cartilage graft (usually rib) is placed to help keep the larynx open (Luft, Wetmore, Tom, Handler, & Potsic, 1989). The success rate of decannulation after laryngotracheoplasty (as required by Frank, see case history, Chapter 1) is 80%.

If all of the criteria for decannulation readiness are met, the child is taken to the recovery room or intensive care setting, placed on

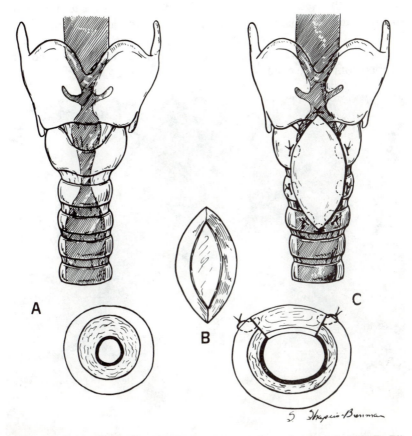

Figure 2-9.   A. Subglottic stenosis, anterior view, and cross section. **B.** Rib graft. **C.** Subglottic stenosis with rib graft interposition, anterior view and cross section.

the caregiver's lap (if the child is physically able to do so), and the tracheostomy tube is removed. **Down sizing** of tracheostomy tubes is not performed as commonly as for adults, because the smaller children's cannulas are much more prone to occlusion and youngsters' airways are smaller and more susceptible to respiratory obstruction. Following decannulation, the stoma is loosely covered with a Band-Aid and the child is observed for 2 hours before transfer to a regular hospital room for 24 hours for observation that the airway is sufficient.

After decannulation, the tracheostomy stoma usually shrinks and closes spontaneously. It may take several days for the stoma to close completely. However, in approximately 50% of the children who have had a tracheostomy tube for longer than 1 year, the tracheostomy tract is **epithelialized** and will not close on its own (Figure 2-10) (Wetmore et al., 1982). In these children, excision of the **tracheocutaneous fistula** must be performed to close the tract (as in Lisa, see Chapter 1). This is usually performed 6-12 months after decannulation to be certain that the child will not need the tracheostomy tube again.

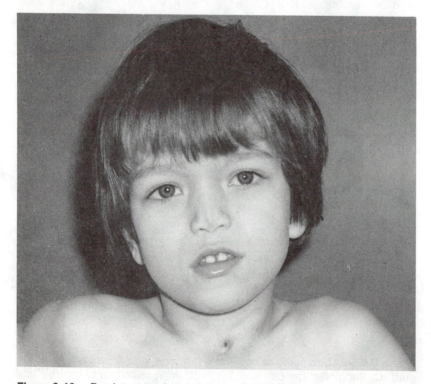

Figure 2-10.   Persistent tracheocutaneous fistula after decannulation.

LARYNGEAL DIVERSION

While **dysphagia** and some minimal **aspiration** are common during the early placement of the tracheostomy tube, aspiration rarely continues. However, in a small group of children who have **neuromuscular disorders** with laryngeal incompetence, chronic aspiration is a serious and potentially life-threatening disorder. Although placement of the tracheostomy tube will allow for suctioning of secretions, the cannula itself will not prevent aspiration. Surgical treatment of chronic aspiration is accomplished through several procedures that, in essence, close the upper respiratory tract from the alimentary tract (DeVito, Wetmore, & Pransky, 1989). The most efficacious of these procedures is **laryngeal diversion**. For the procedure to be performed, aspiration must be documented by a barium swallow, methylene blue study or radio-isotope milk scan (see Chapter 5). The presence of aspiration without significant sequelae is not sufficient justification for diversion. The patient must have severe episodes of recurrent pneumonia and/ or deteriorating pulmonary functions. In such a case, a laryngeal diversion (Figure 2-11) is performed, with the trachea divided and the lower segment sutured to the neck skin, forming a permanent tracheostoma (similar to following laryngectomy).

In laryngeal diversion, the superior tracheal remnant is either sutured closed to make a dead-end pouch or diverted into the esophagus. In either case, the lower airway is completely separate from the alimentary tract and aspiration is impossible. By separating the lower and upper airway, vocalization is also impossible. Although the procedure is theoretically reversible on improvement of the child's neuromuscular condition, the child's status rarely allows for this.

CONCLUSIONS

Surgical management of the child with a tracheostomy requires an understanding of the many reasons for placement of the tracheostomy, as well as expertise in the skills to perform the tracheostomy and associated procedures, such as bronchoscopy, laryngeal diversion, and closure of a persistent tracheocutaneous fistula. Postoperative care includes changing and modifying tracheostomy tubes as the patient's condition requires. The surgical specialist must remain in close contact with the other team members to coordinate efforts to identify and correct conditions that might impede normal speech, language, and feeding development.

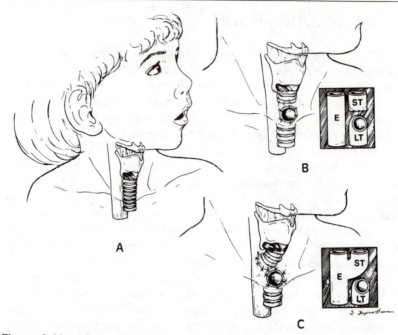

Figure 2-11. Laryngeal diversion. **A.** Normal anatomy. Note relationship between trachea and esophagus. **B.** Laryngeal diversion in which superior trachea (ST) is closed and the lower trachea (LT) is sutured to the neck skin. The esophagus (E) is left untouched. **C.** Laryngeal diversion in which the superior trachea (ST) is diverted into the esophagus (E). The lower trachea (LT) is sutured to the neck skin.

REFERENCES

DeVito, M., Wetmore, R., & Pransky, S. (1989). Laryngeal diversion in the treatment of chronic aspiration in children. *International Journal of Pediatric Otorhinolaryngology, 18,* 139-145.

Handler, S. (1986). Difficult decannulation. In G. Gates (Ed.), *Current therapy in otolaryngology—Head and neck surgery* (pp. 327-329). Philadelphia: B.C. Decker.

Luft, J., Wetmore, R., Tom, L., Handler, S., & Potsic, W. (1989). Laryngotracheoplasty in the management of subglottic stenosis. *International Journal of Pediatric Otorhinolaryngology, 17,* 297-303.

Simon, B., & Handler, S. (1981). The speech pathologist and management of children with tracheostomies. *Journal of Otolaryngology, 10,* 440-448.

Simon, B., & Silverman McGowan, J. (1989). Tracheostomy in young children: Implications for assessment and treatment of communication and feeding disorders. *Infants and Young Children, 1,* 1-9.

Wetmore, R., Handler, S., & Potsic, W. (1982). Pediatric tracheostomy: Experience during the past decade. *Annals of Otology Rhinology and Laryngology, 91,* 628-632.

3

Ventilator Assistance

Stephen Metz

INTRODUCTION

Baby's breath (Gysophilia paniculata) is more than just a delicate flower—it is an essential part of life. From the first moments of extrauterine existence, the child requires a continuous cycling of the respiratory system to sustain that which all so cherish. The mechanisms which ensure this are exquisite in design but fragile in operation. Breathing is so essential to life itself that nature is intolerant of even transient disruption.

This chapter mainly deals with the use of **long-term (chronic) mechanical ventilation (CMV)**, yet is not meant to downplay the importance of nonventilator management in the care of respiratory dysfunction. Actually, the majority of modifications in the daily care of such infants are most likely to be nonventilator. However, there is a large body of experience with oral and even inhalant medication use, including oxygen, given in a variety of settings. There is much less experience with use of CMV. Furthermore, the complications and expenses associated with this modality merit more detailed discussion.

The following topics are discussed in this chapter:

- Normal respiration
- Disorders
- Bronchopulmonary dysplasia
- Mechanical ventilation
- Complication of mechanical ventilation
- Developmental implications
- Location of care

NORMAL RESPIRATION

Normal respiration is largely a matter of "good air in, bad air out." Breathing originates with a signal in the brain which travels down the **phrenic nerve** to activate the **diaphragm.** The diaphragm is a flat muscle attached to the lower ribs; its contraction pulls the ribs downward, which increases the volume of the thorax, sucking in air (inspiration). Air travels from the nose and mouth, down a branching system of tubes (trachea, bronchi, bronchioles), ending in millions of tiny air sacs. These sacs, the alveoli and capillaries, in intimate communication, allow the exchange of oxygen in inspired air with carbon dioxide produced by metabolism. The thinness of alveoli also makes them susceptible to collapse (termed **atelectasis**). **Surfactant**, a substance produced by alveolar cells, lines the sac's inner surface, providing a biochemical scaffolding. Because surfactant is first produced late in gestation, prematurely born infants often lack surfactant and, thus, suffer atelectasis.

DISORDERS

Respiratory failure and thus the need for CMV may occur because of (1) failure to initiate breathing (CNS disease, e.g. **congenital hypoventilation syndrome, encephalopathy**), (2) failure to transmit the signal (phrenic nerve disorders), (3) failure to respond to the signal (diaphragmatic or chest wall disorders), or (4) failure of the target (diseases of the airways or the lungs).

Reasons for a failure to initiate the signal to breathe, originating in the CNS, may range from encephalopathy to brain tumors. The isolated absence of the signal, termed congenital hypoventilation syndrome, is uncommon, but is perhaps the clearest CNS indication for chronic ventilation (Oren, Kelly, & Shannon, 1987). Whether the children whose encephalopathy or other brain injury is so severe as to compromise the very basic brain stem function of breathing should be sustained on CMV is more of an ethical question than a technological one (Farrell & Fost, 1989).

Damage to the phrenic nerve may produce respiratory failure, especially if bilateral; some such traumas may resolve with time, but the extent of recovery is not well predictable early in the course of injury. A patient's inadequate response to the signal to breathe from chest wall deformities distorting the position of the diaphragm or to primary diaphragmatic injury, tends to be insidious in development, and progressive in nature. Severe scoliosis may lead to respiratory insufficiency.

BRONCHOPULMONARY DYSPLASIA

In general, if failure is from a cause other than primary pulmonary disease, mechanical ventilation may be easily accomplished when given reliable equipment, a secure airway, and attentive caregivers.

Lung disease presents a more daunting challenge in both hospital and home. In Schreiner, Donar, and Kettrick (1987), **bronchopulmonary dysplasia (BPD)** was the predominant primary lung disease in pediatric home CMV. Although not all severe chronic lung disease in infants is BPD, BPD provide a model for considering management of complexities.

BPD is defined as a continued need for oxygen beyond 28 days of life, with corresponding X-ray changes such as increases in lung markings. Variations in the susceptible population (born in hospital or transferred), in prenatal status, (e.g., economic status, extent of prenatal care), in neonatal intensive care (NICU) practices (e.g., interfacility variations in target ranges for "acceptable" blood gases), and probably in other as yet unknown factors contribute to a wide variation in the reported incidence of BPD among NICU discharges, ranging from 10-30% of **very low birth weight** infants (Bancalari & Gerhardt, 1986; O'Brodovich & Mellins, 1985). Frank and Lisa, the two children serving as case studies (see Chapter 1), both have BPD.

BPD is an unresolved acute neonatal lung injury; it is usually thought of as unsuccessful resolution of **hyaline membrane disease**, the surfactant-deficiency disease of infants born prematurely. Recognized causes of BPD include **prematurity**, prolonged mechanical ventilation, and high oxygen use; there are also a number of other reputed causes (Bancalari & Sosenko, 1990). Other neonatal pulmonary diseases, such as cytomegalovirus infection or diaphragmatic hernias may produce a clinical picture indistinguishable from garden-variety BPD.

Dysplasia is denoted by microscopically visible changes in the lining of the airway. Infants with BPD often suffer from failure to thrive because of the increased work of breathing through altered airways. On chest X-ray, the picture varies from a mild increase in lung markings to diffuse fibrosis (Figure 3-1).

The recent availability of exogenous (artificial or of animal origin) surfactant for administration to prematurely born infants, before or

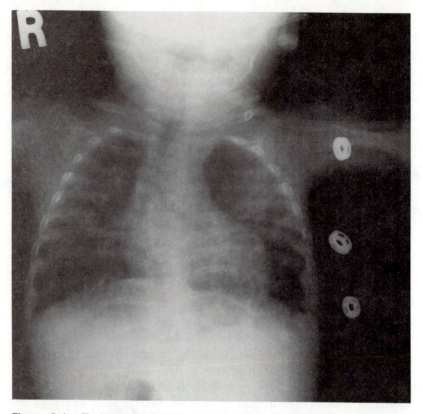

Figure 3-1. Typical portable X-ray picture of a stable BPD patient. Note generalized increase in lung markings.

with the first breath or later as a "rescue" measure, is expected to reduce the severity of hyaline membrane disease and thus the incidence of BPD (Hennes, Lee, Rimm, & Shapiro, 1991). However, while studies indicate that a reduced severity of hyaline membrane disease is evident, a reduced incidence of BPD has not yet been shown (Long et al., 1991). Thus, it is not yet clear whether there will be less BPD in the future or simply a shift to BPD in survivors of lower gestational age than previously viable.

The prognosis for BPD is guardedly good, though certainly dependent on severity in a given patient. If the problems can be effectively treated and growth can be sustained, time will allow remodeling of the patient's airways. However, treatment is often a quite extensive (and of course, expensive) process, sometimes spanning years. Unsuccessful management of chronic lung disease will predictably lead to possibly terminal **pulmonary vascular hypertension** and **cardiomegaly.**

MECHANICAL VENTILATION

The essential function of the respiratory system is the exchange of gases consumed by metabolic processes with those produced by the same processes; **respiratory failure** is inadequacy in the exchange. **Acute respiratory failure** is the sudden inability to accomplish adequate gas exchange. The condition requires support by mechanical ventilation to sustain life. **Chronic respiratory failure** is said to be present when that support extends beyond 28 days. As the specific treatment for respiratory failure, mechanical ventilation has earned a secure place in acute care medicine, and a large portion of patients in surgical, medical, cardiac, pediatric, and neonatal intensive care units need to receive mechanical ventilation. This chapter provides basic familiarity with mechanical ventilation; readers are referred to Mallory and Stillwell (1991), who have prepared an excellent review of CMV and provide a logical framework and summary of published experience with CMV in pediatrics.

Negative Pressure Ventilators

Negative pressure ventilators exert suction on the outside of the thorax, inducing chest expansion. Just as in normal respiration, the reduced intrathoracic pressure accompanying this increased volume induces a flow of air into the lungs. Expiration is accomplished by natural elastic recoil when the suction ceases.

Negative pressure ventilation is the most physiologic form of ventilatory support and, accordingly, has the fewest complications, especially those causing lung damage (Splaingard, Frates, Jefferson, Rosen, & Harrison, 1983). However, these ventilators are cumbersome because suction must be maintained for half the cycle. Although this method does have the advantage of not requiring a **tracheostomy,** there are only a few models available and customization is necessary because of changes with growth, and they cannot provide 24-hour support (especially during sleep). The iron lung is a prime example of the tank-type negative pressure ventilator. More recently, cuirass ventilators, utilizing a moldable thoracic shell, have allowed for patient mobility (O'Leary, King, Leblanc, Moss, Liebhaber, & Lewiston, 1979).

Positive Pressure Ventilators

Positive pressure ventilators, by far the most common type of ventilator, are the focus of most of the remaining discussion. Positive pressure ventilators work by forcing air (positive pressure) into the lungs; elastic recoil provides for expiration. This ventilator requires a secure pathway into the lungs, provided by a tube in the nose or mouth in an acute situation or a tracheostomy if long-term ventilation is expected. Positive pressure ventilation also allows greater ease in administering increased concentrations of oxygen and flexibility in tailoring the support. Table 3-1 lists descriptive terms encountered in the use of positive pressure mechanical ventilators.

Types

Conceptually, if not entirely precisely, there are two major types of positive pressure ventilators, classified by which of two key parameters—volume or pressure—are set by the machine. **Volume ventilators** allow the operator to set a desired tidal volume that the machine will deliver to generate the pressure required to accomplish this, up to preset or adjustable limits which cause alarms and depressurization. **Pressure ventilators** allow the operator to set the pressure at which air will be forced into the lungs, allowing the compliance of the lungs to determine the tidal volume delivered. With the exception of a few versatile ventilators largely restricted to intensive care units, most ventilators are either volume or pressure types.

Another important distinction between ventilators is the state of airflow in the ventilator tubing between machine breaths. Continuous-flow ventilators produce a steady air supply at the child's airway, awaiting a spontaneous breath; intermittent-flow ventilators require patient effort to draw air through the intake hose back to the ventilator. The high flow rates of continuous-flow ventilators are usually no problem in the hospital, but preclude portability. Often the difference between the types becomes evident as one tries to transition a patient to a portable ventilator, which are always intermittent-flow.

Breath Design

Saying simply that a positive pressure ventilator forces air into the lungs belies the complexity with which that breath can be designed, but such creativity is usually inapplicable to CMV. There are four principal variables (three are set, one is either set or measured) defining the primary characteristics of the delivered positive pressure breath and best describing the extent of ventilator support—together the variables constitute the ventilator prescription.

Mode.   The first option is how the ventilator operates ("cycles") in concert with the patient's effort, termed **mode.** Options

TABLE 3-1. Seven attributes of positive pressure ventilators.

ATTRIBUTES	CHARACTERISTICS
1. Movability	Stationary Portable
2. Power Sources	Electrical, with/without battery Electrical, plus pneumatic (requires source of pressurized air)
3. Airflow generation	Piston Bellow Bags
4. Coordination with patient breath (Mode)	Assist—spontaneous patient effort triggers machine breath Control—machine cycles, without regard to patient activity, at preset time intervals Intermittent—patient may trigger machine, and breath between machine breaths; machine will cycle if no patient breath in specified time interval; (may be synchronized with patient effort, i.e., synchronized intermittent mandatory ventilation-SIMV)
5. Positive pressure generation	Pressure—PIP set; tidal volume determined by respiratory compliance Volume—inspiratory tidal volume set; PIP dependent on respiratory compliance
6. Inspiration termination regulation	Time limited—after preset time (determined by I:E ratio) Pressure limited—after preset pressure (PIP) reached Volume limited—after preset volume delivered by machine Flow limited—after preset critical flow rate reached
7. Pressure maintenance in inspiration tubing between machine breaths	Continuous flow—pressurized air near patient Intermittent flow—air in tubing at atmospheric pressure; to take breath, patient must inspire against demand valve (sensitivity may be variable)

include "assist" (ventilator delivers breath only when patient initiates a breath), "control" (ventilator cycles irrespective of patient activity), or a mix of the two. Some ventilators have mechanisms to sense a child's inspiratory effort, and use the feedback information to trigger itself in step with the patient's rhythm (**synchronized intermittent mandatory ventilation [SIMV]**). The sensitivity—the effort needed to trigger such a machine breath—may also vary. SIMV is generally the preferred mode for patients able to initiate some breaths.

Rate. The next consideration is **rate**—simply the number of breaths the machine is to deliver in 1 minute. For practical purposes, this rarely exceeds a setting of 30, and even for quite serious situations, rates greater than 80, while possible, are rarely required. High frequency ventilation, with rates of 60-3,000, is experimental. The difference between the rate provided by the machine and breathing the patient might spontaneously manage without CMV is compensated by the ventilator capacity to deliver a breath deeper than the patient is likely to be able to self-inhale.

Pressure.   The third parameter that (by definition) is preset in pressure ventilators and measured in volume ventilators is **pressure.** Actually, there are two pressures of interest—a **peak inspiratory pressure (PIP)** and **positive end expiratory pressure (PEEP)**, a pressure at the end of the expiratory cycle. As the names imply, PIP is the peak of pressure during inspiration and PEEP is the small pressure at the end of expiration generated by resistance in the airway, particularly at the vocal cords, which typically measures about 2 cm H_2O. These pressures are commonly recorded as PEEP/ PIP. Delivering PEEP with a portable ventilator usually requires an additional device, attached to the outside of the machine.

Concentration.   Finally, the **concentration** of oxygen in the delivered breath can vary from room air (21%) to maximal (100%). Oxygen may be delivered by a variety of devices (See Table 3-2). Oxygen concentrations may need to be increased during some specific interventions for a child, such as stress of daily cares or the exertion needed for physical therapy. With pulse oximetry, desaturations can be quickly seen and responded to. For example, Frank at 6 months old had a ventilator prescription reading "IMV 15-pres 25/6-30%." Translated, this means that Frank was being sustained on a positive pressure ventilator, in an intermittent man-

TABLE 3-2. Comparison of oxygenation devices.

TYPE	ADVANTAGE	DISADVANTAGE
Cylinder	Readily available Relatively inexpensive Portable	Heavy (E cylinder 15 lb., about 5 hrs at 2 LPM) Remote torpedo hazard
Liquid	Portable Home & travel supplies interchangeable Fairly discrete (portable—11 lbs., about 8 hrs. at 2 LPM)	Expensive—not always covered by insurance Some evaporative loss at low flow rates
Concentrator	No deliveries needed	Electricity needed (cost = approx. $200 monthly) Not portable Need back-up in case of power failure

datory ventilatory mode (sensing his breaths so as not to compete with them), at a rate of 15 breaths per minute, with a PIP (peak inspiratory pressure) of 25 cm H_2O, a positive end expiratory pressure of 6, and with an O_2 concentration of 30%. Three months later, after successful transition to a portable ventilator, Frank's orders read "IMV 10-TV 110-PEEP 6-25%," meaning Frank had a positive pressure ventilator (in this case, portable), with the volume (rather than the PIP) set, IMV mode at a rate of 10 breaths per minute, and a PEEP of 6 cm H_2O, with oxygen set at 25%. In general, the higher the numbers in each of the categories, the worse the condition requiring treatment.

Continuous Positive Airway Pressure

Continuous positive airway pressure (CPAP) is the imposition of an expiratory resistance that creates positive pressure throughout the cycle. It can be delivered by a ventilator with a rate set at zero (hence, no breaths actually delivered, only line pressure), or by connecting the patient's airway to circuitry creating the resistance. Positive pressure ventilation via a nasal mask has been used in adults with nocturnal hypoventilation (Kerby, Mayer, & Pingleton, 1987).

Ventilator Models

There are many stationary ventilators available that are well described in standard respiratory care texts (Barnes & Libson, 1988; Burton & Hodgkin, 1984). There is a much more limited selection of portable ventilators. There are no important differences among the four that are readily available. Portable ventilators operate on AC current, with battery backup. The built-in battery in portable ventilators typically has a life of about 1 hour; standard gel cells last 8-12 hours, and acid (marine) batteries last 16-20 hours. All ventilator batteries can be recharged.

COMPLICATIONS OF MECHANICAL VENTILATION

Positive pressure ventilation can lead to a number of complications, some obvious and others subtle. Most involve **barotrauma**, which is the effect of forcing air at supraphysiologic pressures through often young and damaged airways. The dramatic complications of air accumulation in unwanted areas (pulmonary interstitial emphysema, pneumothorax, pneumomediastinum, and pneumopericardium) are fortunately rare in CMV. More subtle complications can arise as an effect on cardiac function, particularly as PEEP rises.

More insidious complications are changes induced in the large airways, where barotrauma transforms normal ciliated columnar epithelium to a squamous variety; this has already been noted as a cause of BPD. Thus the treatment of severe BPD requires use of actual causative agents—ventilation and increased inspired oxygen concentration. The trick in providing such care is to maintain growth for weaning from the treatment.

Infection

Airway surface damage caused by barotrauma or high inspired oxygen concentration makes the surface more inviting to pathogens. A tracheostomy tube, which bypasses upper airway defenses, places the child receiving ventilator assistance more at-risk to infection. The most common cause of rehospitalization for the CMV patient is a lower respiratory tract infection. Marginal nutrition and relative antibody deficiency make this more likely (Lederman, 1989).

Distinguishing viral from bacterial pathogens is not always possible, although panels of several common viral pathogens (influenza A & B, parainfluenza, adenovirus, and respiratory syncytial virus [RSV]), may be helpful. A particular pathogen to be feared is RSV. Specific anti-RSV therapy is available, though controversial.

It is usual to isolate bacteria from tracheostomy secretions of patients on mechanical ventilation; the significance of the finding relies on the entire clinical picture. A laboratory finding of copious white blood cells accompanying the organisms is incriminating, but even that may be seen in a patient who is otherwise quite stable and who would likely not benefit from aggressive antimicrobial therapy. Antibiotics administered by inhalation may be a reasonable course in treating localized airway infection.

Lastly, the water used to humidify ventilator circuitry can harbor pathogens that can then be delivered directly to the trachea and lungs. Outbreaks of nosocomial illness constantly threaten intensive care units. Also, water can accumulate in the tubing and presents at least a remote drowning hazard.

Endotracheal Tube

One "complication," not really caused by the ventilator and actually occurring before attachment to the ventilator, is misplacement of an endotracheal tube. It is easy to insert such a tube into the esophagus. However, even if one is successful in inserting the tube into the trachea, there is still a risk that a long tube enthusiastically inserted may enter the right mainstem bronchus, which is in a more direct path than that of the left. Entrance into the right main stem bronchus largely excludes aeration of the left lung and even the right upper lobe bronchi. Such differential inflation is occasionally exploited in situations of localized right middle or lower lobe collapse, but is otherwise rarely helpful.

Oxygen

Oxygen, so necessary for life, also has distinct toxicity. Average humans receiving 24 hours of pure oxygen (F_1O_2 100%) complain of pain, which becomes more intense by 48 hours; continued administration may be fatal (Burton, 1984). The neonate enjoys some protection from oxygen toxicity, but long-term administration of greater than 40% oxygen may cause impairment in respiratory function, probably as a result of energetic toxic free radical molecules. Vitamin E, a scavenger of such free radicals, enjoyed brief popularity in prevention of BPD, but early enthusiasm has waned.

Mechanical Failure

An essential component of ventilator construction is an alarm system for operational monitoring of the unit. By sensing interaction with the patient (e.g., excessive volumes needed to reach a preset pressure, a leak in the system), the system monitors the patient's status and alarms alert caretakers to abnormalities. Depending on the machine, some limits are variable, others fixed. Failure of the ventilator to respect preset limits and sound alarms appropriately is uncommon but potentially lethal. Obviously, failure of the power source or oxygen supply can have fatal results.

The ventilator is connected to the patient by at least two tubes—one for the inspiratory flow, one for the expiratory flow. Additionally, often a third, stiffer tube is used to measure pressures. Air moves in and out of these tubes according to pressures, so that a positive pressure prevents expired air from re-entering the ventilator. The inspiratory (often blue) and expiratory (white) tubes are typically corrugated, to allow expansion with the respiratory cycle. The volume of air and the pressure lost in filling this tubing must be included in setting up the ventilator. The tubes are commonly fitted with traps to catch excess moisture.

Potential leaks in a system require constant vigilance. Tubes can become disconnected, especially with active children and especially at the intersection of a relatively heavy cluster of tubes attached to an often too small neck. Changing the type of tracheostomy is sometimes helpful in correcting this. Some leakage is expected with uncuffed tracheostomy tubes that are preferred as less injurious to airways and more amenable to speech. Mallory and Stillwell (1991) provide guidelines on determining leakage tolerances.

A Final Consideration

A final word is needed about ventilators and the care of children requiring them—not a complication, but a consideration. The overall health of the child, especially the underlining respiratory health, will determine the child's level of success with CMV. Strength and endurance are limited by respiratory function, and the greater the need for supportive ventilation, the greater the expectation that comprehensive habilitation will be compromised by respiratory impairment, even when blood gasses are corrected to "normal."

LOCATION OF CARE

With success in stabilizing respiratory failure, a new group of children has emerged: those who survive the acute situation, but progress to a chronic respiratory failure, requiring long-term ventilator assistance. It is ironic that the CMV patient should be considered a "new" problem, because the first large-scale success with ventilators were the "iron lungs," used for extended support of polio victims.

Because they dramatically support an essential, vital function, ventilators are usually confined to intensive care units. The crowding of intensive care units with CMV patients extends to the very young. A cross-sectional survey of NICU facilities in North Carolina—one of a number of areas reporting a shortage of such beds—found 38% of NICU beds occupied by patients 31 days of age or older; 25%, 13%, and 8% of the NICU population were receiving CMV at greater than 31, 61, and 91 days, respectively (Stiles, Metzguer, O'Hale, & Cefalo, 1991).

Although the usual goal of every hospital admission is a discharge to the home, continued reliance on mechanical ventilation, even with a relatively stable medical profile otherwise, presents major difficulties to both hospital and home. Yet, if the child's medical conditions are fairly stable, the family is willing and able, and supportive funding is available, such care can be safely provided at home. (See Chapter 10 for a detailed discussion of these issues.) The American Thoracic Society provides published standards relating to home ventilator care for children (Eigen & Zander, 1990).

To help the child and family with the transition from the acute care setting to the community, "transitional" settings have emerged.

Transitional settings are intermediate care facilities either in continuity with NICUs or in freestanding facilities. The goals of transitional settings include ensuring medical stability, educating the family, and mobilizing the resources necessary for a safe discharge home. (See Chapters 10, 11, and 13 for discussions of these issues.) A transitional setting also provides an opportunity to assess other, especially neurodevelopmental, aspects of the child and family's new situation—both often obscured in the glare of the acute situation.

DEVELOPMENTAL IMPLICATIONS

Speech

Ventilators allow for the same forces involved in natural speech—passive chest recoil expelling air from the lungs—but on a rigid basis, not accommodating the cadences of speech. (The discussion in Chapter 6 is pertinent to these issues.) Further, the volume of air needed to provide strength to the voice may be limited, particularly with restrictive lung disease. Most importantly, the usual path of air exiting from the lungs in a patient with a tracheostomy is through the tracheostomy (the path of least resistance), which bypasses the vocal cords; thus little flow can be modulated to produce speech.

Swallowing

A tracheostomy can lead to swallowing difficulties because pressure from air forced through a tracheostomy is directed mainly to the lungs, but mouth pressures may well also increase in the process. Thus, the normal reflexes closing the airway during swallowing lack the usual cues of in and out air flow, because the air flow is below the usual sensing points. **Aspiration** is a common problem in orally fed children receiving ventilator assistance. Less acute but even more common is difficulty in handling normal oral secretions. This vexing problem may be partially addressed with agents decreasing secretions, such as atropine or glycopyrrolate, but no totally satisfactory solution has been found. Nasal regurgitation is often seen in children receiving ventilator assistance, presumably caused by inadequate soft palate elevation.

Lifestyle

Beyond the direct physiologic complications of mechanical ventilation, there is a massive encroachment on a normal lifestyle.

The psychological ramifications of absolute dependency on an extra-corporeal device may be devastating in an adult—though infant health care providers often wish they could impart some sense of fear as children blithely disconnect themselves.

Mobility is a major lifestyle issue, especially if the child's neuromuscular and cognitive skills would otherwise allow such. Although extraordinary tubing lengths have been used, there is progressive loss of air pressure and volume as tubing length increases. The attachment of tubing to a tracheostomy is a large mass that the child cannot comfortably lie down on. An infant's prone skills will likely be delayed until there is enough maturity to lift not only the head but also the neck and the tracheostomy encumbrances as well.

CONCLUSIONS

The medical management of the child with chronic pulmonary disease is complex. Inadequate ventilation will likely require CMV, usually positive-pressure if there is primary pulmonary disease, possibly negative pressure if there is only a neuromuscular disorder. Bronchopulmonary dysplasia is one of the primary conditions giving rise to the need for mechanical ventilation. Although most often performed in acute care settings, mechanical ventilation can also be provided in rehabilitation settings and in the home.

REFERENCES

Bancalari, E., & Gerhardt, T. (1986). Bronchopulmonary dysplasia. *Pediatric Clinics of North America, 33,* 1-23.

Bancalari E., & Sosenko, I. (1990). Pathogenesis and prevention of neonatal chronic lung disease: Recent developments. *Pediatric Pulmonology, 8,* 99-116.

Barnes, T.A., & Lisbon, A. (Eds.). (1988). *Respiratory care practice.* Chicago: Year Book Medical Publishers.

Burton, G.G. & Hodgkin, J.E. (Eds.). (1984). *Respiratory care: A guide to clinical practice* (2nd ed.). Philadelphia: J.B. Lippincott Co.

Eigen, H., & Zander, J. (1990). Home mechanical ventilation of pediatric patients. *American Review of Respiratory Diseases, 141,* 258-259.

Farrell P., & Fost N., (1989). Long-term mechanical ventilation in pediatric respiratory failure: Medical and ethical considerations. *American Review of Respiratory Diseases, 140,* 836-840.

Hennes H.M., Lee M.B., Rimm A.A., & Shapiro D.L. (1991). Surfactant replacement therapy in respiratory distress syndrome: Meta-analysis of clinical trials of single-dose surfactant extracts. *American Journal of Diseases of Children, 145,* 102-104.

Kerby, G.R., Mayer, L.S., & Pingleton, S.K. (1987). Nocturnal positive pressure ventilation via nasal mask. *American Review of Respiratory Diseases, 135,* 738-740.

Lederman, H.M., Metz, S.J., Zuckerbert, A.L., & Loughlin, G.M. (1989). Antibody deficiency complicating severe bronchopulmonary dysplasia. *Pediatric Pulmonology, 7,* 52-54.

Long, W., Thompson, T., Sundell, H., Schumacher, R., Volberg, F., & Guthrie, R. (1991). Effects of two rescue doses of a synthetic surfactant on mortality rate and survival without bronchopulmonary dysplasia in 700- to 1350-gram infants with respiratory distress syndrome. *Journal of Pediatrics, 118,* 595-605.

Mallory, G.B., & Stillwell, P.C. (1991). The ventilator dependent child: issues in diagnosis and management. *Archives of Physical Medicine and Rehabilitation, 72,* 43-55.

O'Brodovich, H.M., & Mellins, R.B., (1985). Bronchopulmonary dysplasia. *American Review of Respiratory Diseases,* 694-709.

O'Leary, J. King, R., Leblanc, M., Moss, R., Liebhaber, M., & Lewiston, N. (1979). Cuirass ventilation in childhood neuromuscular disease. *The Journal of Pediatrics, 94,* 419-421.

Oren, J., Kelly, D.H., & Shannon, D.C. (1987). Long-term follow-up of children with congenital central hypoventilation syndrome. *Pediatrics, 80,* 375-380.

Schreiner, M.S., Donar, M.E., & Kettrick, R.G. (1987). Pediatric home mechanical ventilation. *Pediatric Clinics of North America, 34,* 47-60.

Splaingard, M.L., Frates, Jr., R.C., Jefferson, L.S., Rosen, C.L., & Harrison, D.M. (1983). Home negative pressure ventilation: report of 20 years of experience in patients with neuromuscular disease. *Archives of Physical Medicine and Rehabilitation, 66,* 239-242.

Stiles, A., Metzguer, K., O'Hale, A., & Cefalo, R. (1991). Characteristics of neonatal intensive care unit patients in North Carolina: a cross-sectional survey. *Pediatrics, 87,* 903-908.

SECTION III

DEVELOPMENTAL INTERVENTIONS

4

Management of Physical and Neurodevelopmental Concerns

Lisa A. Kurtz, Michelle J. Davis, and Meg Stanger

INTRODUCTION

This chapter reviews the incidence, characteristics, and management of motor delays and deficits associated with long-term tracheostomies in children, with emphasis on the neonate through toddler. Additionally, this chapter describes the medical precautions that must be observed by all health care professionals providing services to children with tracheostomies. The following topics are covered:

- Motor deficits commonly associated with long-term tracheostomy
- Prerequisite training required to safely implement treatment with children who are ventilator-assisted
- Assessment and treatment considerations relevant to functional adaptation in a variety of environmental settings, including the neonatal intensive care unit (NICU), home, and school

MOTOR DEFICITS ASSOCIATED WITH LONG-TERM TRACHEOSTOMIES

Medical advances in the past decade have resulted in more children surviving serious medical conditions leading to **long-term**

tracheostomies, many of whom may benefit from physical and occupational therapy services for improvement of functional motor and adaptive developmental skills. Although this population was once only rarely encountered by therapists outside of the highly specialized environment of the intensive care unit (ICU), it is increasingly common for therapists to encounter children assisted by technology in home care, early intervention, and school-based practices.

Chronic respiratory failure leading to tracheostomy and ventilator assistance in infants and children may occur as a complication of a wide variety of diseases or disabilities, as summarized in Table 4-1 (Mallory & Stillwell, 1991; Simon & Silverman McGowan, 1989). It seems logical, then, that the motoric abilities of children with long-term tracheostomies are as varied as the underlying medical conditions precipitating surgery. However, the largest number of infants and young children with long-term tracheostomies are very premature infants with chronic lung disease secondary to **bronchopulmonary dysplasia (BPD).** Both Lisa and Frank (see Chapter 1) received their tracheostomies secondary to BPD, although each had very different developmental outcomes. Als et al. (1986) report that approximately 30% of infants with birthweights less than 1,500 g and 70% of infants with birthweights less than 1,000 g require mechanical ventilatory assistance.

Long-term tracheostomy in low birth weight premature infants has been associated with a variety of neurodevelopmental, behavioral, and physical sequelae (Schreiner, Downes, Kettrick, Ise, & Volt, 1987; Sehnal & Palmeri, 1989; Singer et al., 1989). Characteristic developmental concerns of these children are similar to those for children with other chronic medical conditions resulting in prolonged hospitalization, decreased movement and environmental exploration, and decreased caregiver-child interaction. Delayed acquisition of developmental milestones, abnormal muscle tone and movement patterns, vision impairment, feeding difficulties, and behavior disorders are common. Preterm infants typically demonstrate **hypotonia,** with severity relating to gestational age. Also, they lack the advantage of a constricted intrauterine environment that is helpful in the development of flexion patterns. The combined effects of intrinsic hypotonia, prolonged supine positioning without mature antigravity postural reactions, and the effects of life-sustaining medical equipment often reinforce exaggerated extension patterns of the neck, trunk, and extremities (Sweeney, 1985). Several characteristic positional deformities, including **doliocephaly** (flattened, narrow,

TABLE 4-1. Common diseases and conditions associated with pediatric tracheostomy.

REASON FOR TRACHEOSTOMY	DISEASE/CONDITION
Congenital or Acquired Airway Abnormalities	Bronchopulmonary Dysplasia Congenital Heart Disease **Craniofacial Anomalies** **Subglottic Stenosis** **Tracheoesophageal Anomalies** **Tracheomalacia**
Central Nervous System Disorders	Brain Stem or Posterior Fossa Tumor Congenital Central Alveolar Hypoventilation (Ondine's Curse) **Epiglottis** Spina Bifida with Arnold-Chiari Malformation Spinal Cord Trauma (C-4 and above) Spinal Muscular Atrophy (e.g., Werdnig-Hoffmann Disease) Viral Encephalitis
Disease Affecting Respiratory Muscles	Congenital Thoracic Cage Anomalies Congenital Myopathies Duchenne's Muscular Dystrophy

elongated head shape), **torticollis,** external tibial torsion, external rotation deformities at the hips or shoulders, and decreased depth of the rib cage, may result from prolonged supine positioning and decreased neck and trunk mobility secondary to bulk of the tracheostomy tube (Semmler, 1989). Furthermore, physical attachment to tracheostomy tubing and to other medical monitoring equipment interferes with the child's capacity for independent mobility and exploration and poses an obstacle to achieving independence in daily activities.

Although premature infants with chronic lung disease secondary to BPD represent the largest number of children requiring **mechanical ventilation,** other children may require ventilatory assistance as a result of respiratory muscle failure from brain stem, spinal cord, or peripheral nervous system disease. The epidemiology of medical events leading to prolonged ventilator assistance in children is reviewed here to remind physical and occupational therapists of the scope of tracheostomy-associated disabilities that may require (re)habilitative management.

Viral encephalitis, posterior fossa tumors, and complications of spina bifida resulting from the Arnold-Chiari malformation account for most childhood disorders of the brain stem leading to mechanical ventilation.

Trauma resulting in high cervical spinal cord injuries, or a vertebral defect affecting diaphragm, abdominal, and intercostal muscle innervation may also predispose for prolonged mechanical ventilation.

Mechanical ventilation may also be beneficial for the infant or young child with a neuromuscular disease such as Werdning-Hoffmann disease, myotonic dystrophy, or congenital myopathies, and during the later stages of Duchenne's muscular dystrophy. The use of prolonged mechanical ventilation to extend life expectancy in children with progressive neuromuscular disease is a controversial issue that must be conducted only after consideration of the family's wishes and the potential quality of life for the child; however, many children with congenital neuromuscular disease have typical intelligence and may lead fairly independent lives at home and at school with the use of assistive technology.

When tracheostomy is required secondary to a primary central nervous system (CNS) disorder or muscle disease, therapists may employ traditional (re)habilitative methodologies with relatively little adaptation. Early therapy goals might include prevention of skin breakdown and **contractures,** maintenance of respiratory status through postural drainage along with coughing and breathing exercises, strengthening of remaining musculature, and assistance in achieving the highest level of independence possible in daily activities.

PRINCIPLES OF MANAGEMENT

Roles of Physical and Occupational Therapists

Children with mechanical ventilation needs present as a varied population typically requiring the services of many disciplines including, physician specialists, nurses, social workers, psychologists, and therapists. For these children to optimally progress they must be managed through coordinated team effort rather than by fragmented individual services. It is easy for family members as well as professional caregivers to become confused and overwhelmed by the input of the many professionals involved in care of the child. Some children may benefit from a **transdisciplinary** service provision model, in which one team member assumes primary responsibility for communication of treatment recommendations; this can be especially helpful during the initial ICU stay, with one therapist acting as a consultant to the critical care staff on positioning, splinting, exercises, and developmental support.

Role boundaries between physical and occupational therapists tend to be particularly difficult for caregivers to understand, because the two disciplines share similar educational preparation, tend to hold congruent philosophies regarding approaches to intervention, and may possess similar levels of skill in the use of certain specialized therapeutic techniques. Often, the role of physical and occupational therapists within a particular agency is influenced by the philosophy of that agency along with ability to recruit experienced pediatric specialists (Kurtz & Scull, in press).

Both physical and occupational therapists assess and treat children with a variety of developmental, musculoskeletal, neuro-muscular, and cardiopulmonary disorders. **Physical therapy** deals with gross motor skill, balance, and posture in relationship with children's ability to be mobile within the environment. **Occupational therapy** addresses fine motor development, cognitive and perceptual maturation, and psychosocial adjustment in helping the children to develop functional skills needed for play, self-care, and school performance. Both disciplines use play as the primary medium for achieving therapy goals and may employ similar strategies and techniques for positioning, splinting, exercise, and neurodevelop-mental facilitation.

Therapist Competencies

When first approaching treatment for the infant or child with a tracheostomy, it is helpful to remember that basic principles of therapeutic management follow traditional frames of reference for developmental disabilities and will, therefore, be familiar to ex-perienced pediatric therapists. However, an additional set of skills and knowledge is required to safely, confidently, and effectively deliver care in the presence of the complex medical and technolog-ical needs of this population. Therapists who work with children receiving ventilator assistance must employ strict infection control procedures, be able to predict and recognize signs of physiologic distress in children, and must be trained in basic procedures for manipulating such equipment as ventilators, cardiac and respiratory monitors, and feeding tubes. This expanded repertoire is crucial in optimizing the children's developmental potential and ensures there is little risk of harming the child while delivering therapy.

Pediatric clinicians agree that treatment of the neonate, whether ventilated or not, should not be attempted by an entry level therapist, but requires an advanced level of clinical competence (Anderson & Auster-Liebhaven, 1984; Campbell, 1986; Sweeney, 1990). In 1985, the American Physical Therapy Association (APTA) approved the "Competencies Necessary for Advanced Clinical Competence in Pediatric Physical Therapy Practice," which included a description of competencies for working with medically fragile infants in the NICU (Roberts, 1985). In 1989, the APTA Section on Pediatrics published the "Competencies for the Physical Therapist in the NICU" (Scull & Dietz, 1989). The Commission on Practice of the American Occupational Therapy Association (AOTA) is presently developing a similar document, "Knowledge and Skills for Occupational Therapy in the Neonatal Intensive Care Unit." Each document stresses the need for specialized knowledge in neonatal medicine, assessment of neonates, development of early intervention goals, family empowerment, and consultation as a member of a multidisciplinary team. Knowledge of neonatal physiology and pathophysiology, nature and management of energy expenditure in preterm infants, and the NICU technology and environment is also necessary (Campbell, 1986). Completion of a clinical practicum under the supervision of a pediatric therapist with advanced clinical skill in the NICU is also advocated (Campbell, 1986; Scull & Dietz, 1989; Sweeney, 1990).

Therapeutic Precautions

Pretreatment Preparation

Obtaining a thorough medical history is a prerequisite to safe treatment of any patient, but is especially important for the medically fragile child. Many children with tracheostomies have complex medical needs and therapeutic precautions, with the most common summarized in Appendix 4-A. Before approaching the child, the therapist should review the medical chart and consult with medical and nursing staff regarding any recent changes in medical status or special precautions that may influence the plan of care. The therapist should note the child's baseline behavioral state and physiologic status, including heart and respiratory rate, breathing pattern, and skin color, and should check the placement of leads and tubes and the current settings of all monitors. It may be appropriate for the nurse to attend the initial session to assist with monitoring of the infant's medical response to intervention; this can greatly increase the therapist's confidence and lead to improved clinical observations.

Equipment Considerations

Therapists may feel overwhelmed when first confronted with the variety of technologic equipment used in the care of the child with a tracheostomy. Equipment setups vary from facility to facility and change frequently as technology evolves. Lack of familiarity with the various tubes, monitors, leads, and alarms can result in confusion, panic, and potentially dangerous handling errors. Furthermore, therapists who are ill at ease with equipment are unlikely to skillfully interact with the child. Familiarity with the following types of equipment is needed: ventilator, cardiac and respiratory monitors, feeding apparatus, suction machine, oxygen source, pulse oximeter, and emergency materials.

The Ventilator

Before a therapy session, the therapist should note the type and placement of the tracheostomy and should check the ventilator and monitors for current settings. The child's activity level and skin color should be noted, with suctioning requested, if necessary. The tubing attached to the tracheostomy should be checked for condensation, and any visible fluid emptied before attempting to handle the child.

Therapy activities must be planned to allow sufficient slack in the tubing to prevent **decannulation.** Ease of movement is best if the tubing swivels at the connector. During movement transitions, tubing should be in line with the connector and free of kinks. Disconnected tubing or a kink preventing the passage of air will be signaled by alarms; the problems can be readily corrected by a knowledgeable therapist and do not require nursing assistance. When moving the child, it is extremely important that any condensation in tubing not flow toward the child's throat to cause **aspiration;** therefore, it is necessary to keep the child's head and tracheostomy opening higher than the tubing and to periodically drain water as it collects in the tubing. Accidental aspiration of water calls for immediate notification of nursing staff and suctioning.

The therapist must know that the child may require suctioning more than once during a session, because physical activity may cause an increased flow of secretions. Signs of physiologic distress signaling the possible need for suctioning are presented in Table 4-2.

The Cardiac Monitor

Some children may be placed on a cardiac monitor. It is a good idea to ask the nurse or primary caregiver for the child's typical range of heart rate during activity. Then, note the baseline heart rate prior to treatment and periodically check the monitor during treatment. Cardiac leads are often sensitive to movement, which may set off alarms. Check the lead placement before treatment for replacement, if dislodged. If your actions do not silence alarms and/

TABLE 4-2. Signs of physiologic distress signaling need for suctioning.

SIGNS OF PHYSIOLOGIC DISTRESS

Frightened, scared look
Skin color changes, such as blue tint around lips or nailbeds
Flared nostrils
Fast breathing, or a rattling noise during breathing
Skin draws in around tracheostomy, below ribs, or beneath sternum
Bubbles of mucus around tracheostomy site
Coughing or gagging
Restlessness
Clammy skin
Behavioral changes, such as lethargy or irritability

or the heart rate is not within safe range, the nurse or primary caregiver must be called for intervention.

Feeding Equipment

It is important to know the child's feeding methods and schedule when planning the treatment session. If the child has **gastroesophageal reflux,** it is a good rule of thumb to treat the child 1 hour before, or 1½ hours after a feeding. If the child is fed through a **nasogastric tube**, it is helpful to coil the end of the tube and tape it to the child's clothing to avoid tangling during dynamic treatment and to prevent both child and therapist from accidentally pulling at it. If the child must be treated while the nasogastric feeding tube is running, remember to allow sufficient slack to prevent the tube from dislodging. If the child is fed through a **gastrostomy** or **jejunostomy tube,** such may be taped securely to the child's abdomen.

Physiologic Stress

Care must be taken to grade therapy according to each child's physiologic tolerance, behavioral responsiveness, and neuromuscular capabilities, as well as to minimize physiologic stress that may result from treatment (see Table 4-2). Both preterm and full-term infants demonstrate negative physiologic responses to routine caregiving, including decreased heart and respiratory rates, decreased blood pressure, and skin color changes (Sweeney, 1986). Als (1986) proposes a behavioral organization model assessing the infant's tolerance to handling and to environmental stimuli and stressing the need for physiologic stability before the infant can progress to motoric competence development. Signs that therapy may be too stressful for the child can include changes in autonomic nervous system function, motoric function, or behavioral state.

Infection Control

Infection control precautions cannot be overemphasized in treating the child with a tracheostomy. The medical vulnerability of these children, along with the high probability of contact with secretions, poses risk to the therapist as well as the child. Rigorous hand washing is the best defense against infection. In addition, careful cleansing of all reusable toys and equipment is imperative. Although specific protocols for infection control will vary between facilities, universal precautions are appropriate for all patient contacts. Under universal precautions, blood and certain body fluids are considered potentially infectious for human immunodeficiency virus (HIV), hepatitis B virus, and other blood-borne pathogens. Health care providers are advised to apply barrier precautions if there is any risk of exposure to blood-infected fluids. Because blood may not be visible in feces, therapists should always wear gloves during diaper changes. Also, therapists with open wounds or sores on their hands should wear gloves during patient treatment. Barrier precaution for infection control may include the use of gloves, gown, mask, or goggles. The degree to which precautions are employed is based on clinical judgment as to the likelihood of exposure to potentially infectious secretions. Appendix 4-C outlines specific techniques for hand washing, equipment sanitization, and barrier precautions.

ASSESSMENT AND TREATMENT CONSIDERATIONS

Neonatal Intensive Care Unit (NICU)

Neonatal intervention is a highly specialized area of occupational and physical therapy practice. Therapists choosing to work in a NICU need to have a thorough knowledge of normal and premature infant development, embryology, physiology, functional and anatomical neurology, and issues relating to organization of behavior and mental state control. This chapter highlights the assessment and treatment considerations of the neonate with respiratory complications leading to tracheostomy, but a detailed discussion is beyond its scope.

Much of the literature on the premature infant in the NICU has focused on the negative effects of the environment on behavior and development of the growing infant (Frank, Maurer, & Shepard, 1991; Gottfried, 1985). The rigorous medical intervention required with these infants often results in diffuse sleep states, excessive handling by caregivers, poor positioning, excess exposure to light and noise within the unit, and poorly timed social and caregiving interactions. These behavioral and environmental effects of the NICU nursery can greatly influence the **arterial oxygen saturation** of the infant with respiratory disease, and must be addressed in the overall treatment plan (Als et. al., 1986).

Models of intervention for neonatal care advocate an individualized approach to treatment, based on assessment of each infant's maturity level, integrity of the central nervous system, and behavioral response to intervention (Blanchard, 1990; Sainte-Anne Dargassies, 1977). There are many neurobehavioral evaluations available for assessing and guiding treatment of the neonate, summarized in Appendix 4-B. During assessment, the therapist must be aware of factors that may influence a neonate's behavioral responses, muscle tone, or motoric activity. These can include gestational age, sleep/wake state at the time of testing, physiological stability, and other environmental factors that may have a profound effect on the neonate's performance (Palisano & Short, 1985). The therapist must also be aware of the limited predictive validity of infant neuromotor assessment tools in predicting later developmental outcome (Marx, 1990).

Following assessment, treatment emphasizes a developmental approach that incorporates the following (Anderson & Auster-Liebhaber, 1984):

1. A strong, cohesive team approach to intervention;
2. Positioning and handling to promote normal developmental postural and movement patterns;
3. Selective sensory intervention (visual, auditory, tactile, proprioceptive, vestibular) to promote infant development;
4. Oral-motor assessment and treatment; and
5. Early caregiver involvement in developmental caregiving.

Many infants with tracheostomies seen in the NICU present with a myriad of medical, neuromuscular, or sensory problems requiring (re)habilitative input. However, the infant's tolerance to intervention is of the utmost importance and must drive the aggressiveness of treatment. Therapists must remember at all times that neurodevelopmental intervention must not interfere with the medical treatment needed to sustain life and must guard against placing undue stress on the infant's CNS (Anderson & Auster-Liebhaber, 1984). Infants with severe respiratory compromise, such as Frank (see Chapter 1), must expend a great deal of energy just to survive and have little reserve for environmental or social interaction.

Strong caregiver involvement from the onset of treatment intervention allows for a smoother transition from hospital to home. By sharing developmental information, observing and discussing the infant's behavior with the caregiver, identifying the caregiver's goals, and engaging in mutual problem solving, the therapist can help facilitate the shift from infant-centered care to family focused care within the hospital environment (Stryzewski, 1989). On discharge home, implementation of a therapeutic program requires sensitivity to the family's need to adjust, close coordination with multiple care providers, flexibility in scheduling, and continued attention to safety and infection control precautions (Ahmann & Lipsi, 1991).

Frank

The following hypothetical case story describes early assessment and treatment planning for Frank (see Chapter 1) and is designed to highlight the motor, sensory, and behavioral characteristics of the preterm infant with respiratory complications leading to tracheostomy.

Background

Frank was born at 28 weeks gestation, weighing just under 1,500 g, to a single mother who was an occasional drug abuser. Neonatal complications included BPD, **intraventricular hemorrhage,** and gastroesophageal reflux. He received a tracheostomy and ventilator assistance at 3 months of age.

Frank was referred to rehabilitation at age 6 months (corrected age 3 months). He was tracheostomized and on 40% oxygen, with ventilator settings of 40 breaths per minute. He was fed via nasogastric tube and was beginning to take some formula by bottle with difficulty. Frank's primary nurse reported that Frank became very irritable during routine care, was difficult to console, arched frequently during feeding or when being held, had poor visual regard, and appeared inattentive when awake and restless when asleep.

The major medical equipment used in Frank's care included a positive pressure ventilator, cardiac monitor, feeding pump, and swivel tracheostomy tube. Baseline heart rate was 165-170, and color was pink throughout extremities. Occupational and physical therapy planned an initial joint evaluation session, scheduled 1½ hours postfeeding, to begin treatment planning. It is often advisable to conduct evaluation of the young infant over several short sessions, because the infant's tolerance for activity may be limited and behavioral responses may vary throughout a day.

Observations of Posture at Rest

At the start of the evaluation, Frank was in light sleep in the prone position. Observation prior to handling revealed that posture was characterized by lower extremity extension, upper extremities were abducted with elbows minimally flexed away from the body, head was turned to the right. Slight jerky movements were observed in the extremities, and slight irregularities in breathing pattern were noted. The infant in the isolette next to Frank was undergoing routine care, lights in the nursery were on, and several medical staff members were holding a discussion in the area.

Behavioral State and Sensory Responses

Frank was gently awakened for beginning of handling. He demonstrated fleeting visual fixation and inconsistent visual tracking of the therapist's face or of a brightly colored object. His level of alertness was inconsistent, ranging from glassy-eyed inattentiveness to brief periods of hyperalertness. Response to auditory input was inconsistent, but he easily startled at the sound of a bell and appeared to demonstrate quieting to the sound of a human voice. As he became periodically irritable during the session, he was able to respond with calming to slow rocking and deep, firm touch. Overall, Frank exhibited decreased ability to modulate sleep/wake/ interaction state behaviors. When Frank was placed in a blanket on the therapist's lap, he exhibited frequent postural movements, but continually resisted a semiflexed position and attempted to arch away from the therapist. Heart and respiratory rates remained relatively constant during this portion of the session.

Neuromuscular Status

Frank demonstrated underlying low muscle tone throughout the trunk and extremities, with increased tone during periods of irritability. Postural behavior was worrisome. In prone, Frank attempted to lift his head for brief periods, demonstrating neck hyperextension, lateral rotation, and scapular retraction, along with increased trunk and lower extremity extension. When placed in supine, Frank had difficulty maintaining his head in midline secondary to tracheostomy placement as well as limited muscle control. Minimal spontaneous movements of the extremities or hand-to-mouth movements were noted. His head lagged during pull-to-sit, and he displayed a rounded back and poor midline positioning during supported sitting. He was unable to sustain weight on his feet for more than a few seconds during supported standing and assumed the "high guard" posture with scapular retraction, shoulder elevation, neck hyperextension, elbow flexion, and hand fisting. Handling needed to be interrupted frequently to calm Frank's irritability and slightly irregular breathing patterns. Although his heart rate raised slightly, it remained within "safe" ranges as given by nursing. Calming was achieved when held upright at the therapist's shoulder and when given firm support at the back and buttocks along with slow, firm pats to his upper back. This also seemed to help break up congestion which tended to increase when he cried. At one point, Frank's crying assumed a rattling quality, indicating the need to suction him.

Treatment Planning and Intervention

Based on assessment findings by the physical and occupational therapists, the following goals were established:

1. To provide positioning suggestions to stimulate active flexion of the trunk and limbs, to enhance symmetric posture and midline orientation, and to facilitate smooth antigravity limb movement (Updike, Schmidt, Macke, Cahoon, & Miller, 1986);
2. To provide controlled sensory input designed to facilitate a calm, alert state and to enhance purposeful interaction with the environment (Anderson & Auster-Liebhaber, 1984);
3. To effect short-term change in muscle tone and postural movements through selected sensory input provided through neurodevelopmental handling techniques;
4. To instruct mother and nursing staff in strategies for handling, calming, and developmentally appropriate social interaction; and
5. to provide anticipatory guidance as Frank progresses through developmental stages of learning.

Frank was seen daily for therapy, with occupational and physical therapy on alternating days. The length of each session varied according to Frank's tolerance; a large portion of each treatment session was spent on caregiver education.

Results of Intervention

Initially, treatment focused on increasing Frank's tolerance to handling and position changes, because this was a major obstacle to all interactions. His therapists understood the need to respect the fragility of Frank's immature CNS; he needed to expend a great deal of energy just to survive, and had limited reserve for purposeful environmental interaction. Nevertheless, they felt frustrated that a child with such need for neurodevelopmental treatment could tolerate only minimal handling without risk for adverse physiological reactions. Fortunately, Frank was able to give clear signals when distressed, and this was helpful in identifying exactly what types of sensory input helped him to organize his behavior. His mother's natural instinct was to bounce him, pat him gently on the back, and sing to him when he became upset; however, this only served to increase Frank's irritability. The therapists pointed out Frank's signals of overstimulation, which included yawning, hiccuping, and gaze aversion, demonstrating better ways of introducing calming sensory input. As Frank's mother gained success in reading his cues, she began to feel more confident in her role as a caregiver.

A written positioning program was posted at Frank's bedside to encourage a flexed posture and to provide boundaries to control extraneous movements whether he was resting in prone, supine, or sidelying positions. Because he responded so positively to firm touch, it was suggested that he be kept bundled and positioned with supportive blanket rolls and small bean bags. The prone position is beneficial for many babies because it requires less energy expenditure and promotes increased time in quiet sleep than does the supine position (Masterson, Zuckerm, & Schulze, 1987). It also facilitates tactile input to the face through hand-to-mouth contact, which is difficult to achieve in supine because of limited control of midline hand skills. Caution in positioning of the tracheostomy tube and ventilator tubing is necessary when placing the child in prone. A hammock-like swing covered in lambswool was adapted for Frank by cutting a hole in the side of the hammock to accommodate the tubing; this proved to be a very helpful intervention strategy, because he calmed well to slow movement and neutral warmth.

Once Frank's medical condition began to stabilize and his tolerance to handling improved, he was able to participate in more dynamic intervention designed to increase active movement and to promote adaptation to objects and people in his environment.

TREATMENT OF THE OLDER CHILD

Models of Intervention

Children who require prolonged ventilator assistance may be hospitalized for many months or even years. The obvious disadvantages of confinement in a noisy, often frightening hospital environment, combined with isolation from the primary family unit, can contribute to a number of developmental, behavioral, and social concerns. Therapists should make every effort to expose older children to a range of "normal" social experiences. Caregiver education should emphasize empowerment in making decisions about the child's care. To the extent possible, patients should follow a predictable daily routine of scheduled activities and should have consistent caregivers (Mallory & Stillwell, 1991). Inpatient early intervention programs, community trips and other group treatment programs may be difficult to coordinate, because these tend to require careful safety planning and a high staff-to-patient ratio; however, the potential benefits are well worth the effort.

As the rehabilitation team begins to plan for the child's transition to home and community environments, it is helpful for therapists to be thoroughly familiar with federal and local legislation governing the educational rights of children with or at risk for disabilities, including the Developmental Disabilities Assistance Act Amendments of 1987 (PL 100-146), which includes a definition of assistive technology services, and the Individuals with Disabilities Education Amendments of 1990 (PL 101-236) (see Chapter 9). Community-based therapists with limited experience working with children who are ventilator-assisted should consider establishing a mentorship relationship with a therapist who can offer experience in treating and monitoring the development of this population (Ahmann & Lipsi, 1991).

Treatment of Mobility Concerns

The functional mobility level of children who are ventilator-assisted can range from independent ambulation without assistive devices to dependence on a motorized wheelchair. Methods of assessment for functional mobility and measurements for assistive devices are similar to those for any child receiving therapy services, although it is helpful to know which strollers and wheelchairs can accommodate ventilators and how to deal with tubing.

Ambulatory children may be significantly restricted by the length of their tubing. Sometimes, length of tubing may be increased without compromising respiratory sufficiency, although any such change needs the physician's approval. To limit stepping on or entanglement with the tubing, it may be helpful to pin it to the child's shirt. This allows for slack near the tracheostomy site if the tubing is pulled at a distance farther from the child. Surprisingly, most children quickly become adept at negotiating turns to prevent tangles. Therapists should attempt to be creative in exposing the child to a variety of sensorimotor experiences; with care, children receiving ventilator assistance can have fun on slides, swings, and obstacle courses just as any other child.

Nonambulatory children will require wheelchairs or other seating systems. Some commercially available seating systems and wheelchair models are able to accommodate a tray for a portable ventilator. The therapist should order from a manufacturer that has a manufacturer-installed tray. This will ensure that the tray will accommodate the weight of the ventilator, that the wheelchair is balanced to compensate for the added weight, and that the tray is properly welded to the frame.

MOTOR PERSPECTIVES ON LEARNING TO COMMUNICATE

Children with long-term tracheostomies are at high risk for communicative impairment, especially when the cannula is in place. At the approximate cognitive developmental level of 9 to 15 months, most children are capable of learning symbols and should be evaluated for an augmentative or alternative communication system (Simon & Silverman McGowan, 1989). Numerous options are available, including eye gaze, nonverbal vocalizations, artificial speech using an electrolarynx, gestures, manual sign language, communication boards, or computerized electronic devices (see Chapter 6). The speech-language therapist is responsible for identifying which system or combination of systems is most appropriate for the individual child's specific communication needs and is responsible for training implementation. However, successful use of augmentative and alternative communication systems may be dependent, in part, on the child's motoric ability to access the system. It is in this area that occupational and physical therapists may offer expertise.

Sign Language is a form of augmentative communication frequently taught to young children with tracheostomies with limited or absent vocal abilities. Execution of manual signs requires a variety of motor skills, ranging from gross whole arm movements (e.g., "thank you"), to complex bilateral movement patterns (e.g., "jump"), to refined hand movements incorporating distal isolation (e.g., "medicine"). Occupational therapists can be helpful in determining the child's maturity for performance of component movements and the presence of perceptual or motor planning difficulties that may influence mastery. In some cases, direct treatment of motor delays or deficits is indicated. The therapist may also provide consultation to the speech-language pathologist regarding:

1. Optimal positioning for efficiency in upper extremity control. Most children will attend best when comfortably seated. Some children may require adapted seating to compensate for impaired motor skills. For example, providing trunk support and positioning the scapulas in slight protraction may benefit the child with exaggerated extension and poor midline hand skills.
2. Motor learning strategies appropriate to the child's developmental level and learning style. For example, some children with delayed perceptual skills learn faster when the teacher/ therapist sits next to (instead of facing) the child to avoid mirror-imaging. Some children may benefit from additional visual or tactile cues when first introduced to a new sign. For example, having a glove on one hand may help the child learning a complex two-handed sign.
3. Advice about vocabulary selection. When acceptable alternatives exist, therapists can offer advice about vocabulary selection, assisting in selection of signs that are motorically easier to execute. Dunn (1982) provides an excellent analysis of the motor complexity of various signs. Considerations may include:

   a. The nature of movement in relation to the body (toward or away from the body; toward or away from midline; use of pronated or supinated forearm positions; presence or absence of visual or tactual reinforcement);
   b. Hand usage patterns (unilateral; bilateral and symmetrical; bilateral with dominant/assistive pattern; bilateral/ reciprocal);
   c. Hand shape (whole hand; thumb isolation; index finger isolation; complex isolation); and
   d. Complexity of motor sequences involved in executing the sign.

Alternative communication systems, including those producing synthesized speech, may be appropriate for children with severe oral-motor dysfunction and poor speech intelligibility (Simon & Silverman McGowan, 1989). Selection and training in use of these devices requires a team approach. Occupational and physical therapists can contribute to the process through:

1. Selection and adaptation of seating or other positioning devices optimizing physical access to the device, reducing fatigue, and increasing control for performing repetitive movements;

2. Identification of the most efficient mode of input, such as pointing, eye gaze, or use of switches;
3. Selection and placement of the optimal switch or other input mode; and
4. Functional vision and perceptual assessment in relation to placement of symbol targets.

SELF-CARE SKILLS

As other children, children with long-term tracheostomies should be encouraged to become as independent as possible in all aspects of self- care, including feeding, dressing, personal hygiene, and recreation. Instruction on all self-care skills should begin at the normal developmental age. Because of the medical attention required with a tracheostomy, it is easy for caregivers and others to fall into the habit of performing care for the child long after the youngster is developmentally ready for self-care independence.

Principles of treatment are similar to those for other children with developmental or physical disabilities; however, some accommodations for equipment are wise. For example, clothing should be loose fitting and easy to don and doff. Front-opening shirts that can be buttoned or zippered are practical, and can be left slightly open at the neck to accommodate the tubing.

Assessment and treatment procedures for feeding and oral-motor problems encountered by children with tracheostomies are covered in Chapter 5. However, it is important to recognize how oral-motor difficulties can interfere with self-feeding behaviors and with oral hygiene. Oral defensiveness is common among children with tracheostomies, and may be caused, in part, by decreased tactile-proprioceptive experiences around the mouth. The spoon, cup, toothbrush, and other utensils should be introduced at the developmentally appropriate age, even if the child is not an oral feeder. Serious oral stimulation avoidance behaviors may require specific sensorimotor intervention to decrease tactile hypersensitivity. Inclusion of the child during the family's normal mealtime can help to model self-feeding behaviors, even if the child is not able to manually consume food.

CONCLUSIONS

Children with long-term tracheostomies may present with a wide range of physical, behavioral, and neurodevelopmental concerns requiring (re)habilitative management. Physical and occupational therapists are integral members of the health care team providing coordinated care in the intensive care unit and rehabilitation settings, at home and school. Effective treatment of this population requires familiarity with the special medical and technological needs of medically fragile children, flexibility, collaboration with multiple caregivers, and an advanced level of competency in pediatric intervention. Community-based therapists with limited experience in this area are encouraged to seek mentorship relationships with hospital-based therapists in order to gain confidence with children who are technology-assisted.

REFERENCES

Ahmann, E., & Lipsi, K.A. (1991). Early intervention for technology-dependent infants and young children. *Infants and Young Children, 3(4),* 67-77.

Als, H. (1986). A synactive model of neonatal behavioral organization: A framework for the assessment of neurobehavioral development in the premature infant and for support of infants and parents in the neonatal intensive care environment. *Physical and Occupational Therapy in Pediatrics, 6(3),* 3-53.

Als, H., Lawhon, G., Brown, E., Gibes, R., Duffy, F.H., McAnulty, G., & Blickman, J.G. (1986). Individualized behavioral and environmental care for the very low birth weight preterm infant at risk for bronchopulmonary dysplasia: Neonatal intensive care unit and developmental outcome. *Pediatrics, 78(6),* 1123-1132.

Anderson, J., & Auster-Liebhaber, J. (1984). Developmental therapy in the neonatal intensive care unit. *Physical and Occupational Therapy in Pediatrics, 10(1),* 89-106.

Blanchard, Y. (1990). Intervention in the neonatal intensive care unit: Annotated Bibliography. *Physical and Occupational Therapy in Pediatrics, 10(1),* 13-85.

Campbell, S.K. (1986). Organizational and educational considerations in creating an environment to promote development of high-risk infants. *Physical and Occupational Therapy in Pediatrics, 6(3),* 191-204.

Dunn, M.L. (1982). *Pre-Sign language motor skills.* Tucson, AZ: Communication Skill Builders.

Frank A., Maurer, P. & Shepard, J. (1991). Light and sound environment: A survey of neonatal intensive care units. *Physical and Occupational Therapy in Pediatrics, 11(2),* 27-45.

Gottfried, A.W. (1985). Environment of newborn infants in special care units. In A.W. Gottfried & J.L. Gaiter (Eds.), *Infant stress under intensive care* (pp. 23-54). Baltimore: University Park Press.

Kurtz, L.A., & Scull, S.A. (in press). Rehabilitation for developmental disabilities: Physical therapy and occupational therapy. In M.L. Batshaw

& S.E. Levy (Eds.), *Pediatric clinics of North America: The developmentally disabled child.* Philadelphia: W.B. Saunders Co.

Mallory G.B., & Stillwell, P.C. (1991). The ventilator-dependent child: Issues in diagnosis and management. *Archives in Physical Medicine and Rehabilitation, 72,* 43-55.

Marx, J. (1990). Predictive value of early neuromotor assessment instruments. *Physical and Occupational Therapy in Pediatrics, 9* (4), 69-79.

Masterson, J., Zucker, C., & Schulze, K. (1987). Prone and supine positioning effects on energy expenditure and behavior of low birth weight neonates. *Pediatrics, 80(5),* 689-692.

Palisano, R., & Short, M. (1985). Methods for assessing muscle tone and motor functions in the neonate: A review. *Physical and Occupational Therapy in Pediatrics, 4(11),* 43-55.

Roberts, P. (1985). *Physical therapy advanced clinical competencies: Pediatrics.* [City, State] American Physical Therapy Association Specialty Council.

Sainte-Anne Dargassies, S. (1977). Neurodevelopmental symptoms during the first year of life, Part I: Essential landmarks for each key age. *Developmental Medicine and Child Neurology, 14,* 235.

Schreiner, M., Downes, J., Kettrick, R., Ise, C., & Volt, R. (1987). Chronic respiratory failure in infants with prolonged ventilator dependency. *Journal of the American Medical Association, 258,* 3398-3404.

Scull, S., & Dietz, J. (1989). Competencies for the physical therapist in the neonatal intensive care unit (NICU). *Pediatric Physical Therapy, 1(1),* 11-14.

Sehnal, J.P., & Palmeri, A. (1989). High-risk infants. In P.N. Pratt & A.S. Allen (Eds.), *Occupational therapy for children* (2nd ed.) (pp. 361-381). St. Louis: The C.V. Mosby Co.

Semmler, C. (1989). Positioning and deformities. In C. Semmler (Ed.), *A guide to care and management of very low birthweight infants: A team approach.* Tucson, AZ: Therapy Skill Builders.

Simon, B., & Silverman McGowan, J. (1989). Tracheotomy in young children: Implications for assessment and treatment of communication and feeding disorders. *Infants and Young Children, 1,* 1-9.

Singer, L.T., Kercsmar, C., Legris, G., Orlowski, J.P., Hill, B.P., & Doershuk, C. (1989). Developmental sequelae of long-term infant tracheostomy. *Developmental Medicine and Child Neurology, 31,* 224-230.

Strzyzewski, S. (1989). The transition from NICU to home. American Occupational Therapy Association, Inc. *Sensory Integration Special Interest Section Newsletter, 12(3),* 1-3.

Sweeney, J.K. (1985). Neonates at developmental risk. In D.A. Umphred (Ed.), *Neurological rehabilitation Vol. 3* (pp. 137-164). St. Louis: C.V. Mosby Co.

Sweeney, J.K. (1986). Physiologic adaptation of neonates to neurologic assessment. *Physical and Occupational Therapy in Pediatrics, 6(3),* 155-169.

Sweeney, J.K. (1990). At-risk neonates and infants, NICU management and follow-up. In D.A. Umphred (Ed.), *Neurological rehabilitation,* (2nd ed.) (pp. 183-231). Philadelphia: the C.V. Mosby Co.

Updike, C., Schmidt, R.E., Macke, C., Cahoon, J., & Miller, M. (1986). Positional support for premature infants. *American Journal of Occupational Therapy, 40,* 712-715.

APPENDIX 4-A

Therapeutic Precautions for Medically Fragile Children

1. Ventilator-assisted

Preparation for Therapy

- Obtain history and emergency procedures
- Check current ventilator settings
- Note type and place of tracheostomy, baseline heart and respiratory rate (from monitors), breathing pattern
- Observe activity level and skin color
- Request suctioning if necessary
- Empty water from tubing

Management of Equipment

- Avoid kinking of tubing
- Provide sufficient slack for tubing, especially if child's setup lacks a swivel tracheostomy
- Watch for condensation accumulation in tubing; empty as necessary, and be careful that fluid does not back up into the tracheostomy
- If necessary to release tubing, provide slack, and replace connecting piece quickly
- Have emergency equipment near the child at all times

Physiological Warning Signs

- Color changes
- Exaggerated breathing patterns
- Alteration in heart rate or respiratory rate
- Coughing
- Change in manner (lethargy, irritability)

Special Therapy Precautions

- Straps on adaptive seats or positioning equipment should be snug but not so tight as to reduce adequate lung expansion
- May need to request suctioning midway through treatment because of loosening of mucus during movement
- May see decreased abdominal control, and decreased righting reactions, flexion and rotation
- May see decreased endurance, general decrease in mobility
- Poor midline skills

2. Cardiac Conditions

Preparation for Therapy

- Obtain history regarding precautions and emergency procedures
- Note baseline heart rate and color

Management of Equipment

- Know how to read cardiac monitor
- Ask nurse if child may be removed from monitor during therapy
- Have emergency equipment available at all times

Physiological Warning Signs

- Color changes
- Increased heart and/or respiratory rate, chest retractions, nasal flaring
- Lethargy
- Irritability

Special Therapy Precautions

- Decreased tolerance to prone and activity in general; employ energy conservation principles
- May have decreased proximal stability, poor rotational skills

3. Central Line

Preparation for Therapy

- Obtain history regarding precautions and emergency procedures

Management of Equipment

- Allow slack for tubing when infusion is running; avoid kinking
- Secure tubing to patient when infusion not running
- Have emergency equipment available (sterile gauze, padded hemostat)

Physiological Warning Signs

• Wet dressing or blood stain
• Blood back-up in tubing
• Air bubble in tubing
• Disorientation, pallor, chest pain (may lead to cardiac arrest)

Special Therapy Precautions

• Child may be placed in prone, but avoid pressure to site of insertion
• If child shows any sign of physiologic distress, place on left side with head below heart and begin emergency procedures

4. Gastrointestinal Conditions

Preparation for Therapy

• Obtain history of feeding schedule, type of feeding, presence and reflux, procedures to prevent reflux

Management of Equipment

• Allow sufficient slack to tubes, if feed is running
• Secure loose tubing to prevent from being pulled out
• May need to empty colostomy or jejunostomy bag before session

Physiological Warning Signs

• Formula leaking from tubing (clamp site or skin site)
• NG tube moves in and out
• Increased irritability
• Emesis

Special Therapy Precautions

• May be less active; may resist prone position
• May note decreased tone; may note fatty quality to muscle
• Wearing one-piece playsuit may help child from pulling on abdominal tubes

5. Oxygen via Nasal Cannula

Preparation for Therapy

• Obtain history regarding emergency precautions
• Note skin color, respiratory function, activity level (if applicable)

Management of Equipment

• Allow sufficient slack for tubing
• Assure that nasal prongs are in place

- Monitor pulse oximeter readings
- Monitor level of oxygen in tank

Physiological Warning Signs

- Change in skin color
- Labored breathing, nasal flaring
- Irritability
- Lethargy

Special Therapy Precautions

- Consider requesting an increase in oxygen level during therapy to increase endurance
- May see decreased tolerance for prone position

6. Peripheral IV Line

Preparation for Therapy

- Obtain history regarding effects of medication and emergency procedures
- Ask if restrictive splints/boards may be removed

Management of Equipment

- Allow slack for tubing and to avoid kinking when infusion is running
- Secure tubing to patient when infusion is not running

Physiological Warning Signs

- Leakage of fluid or blood at site of insertion of line

Special Therapy Precautions

- Avoid weight-bearing on extremity distal to site of insertion

7. Seizures

Preparation for Therapy

- Obtain history on type of seizure, effects of medication, activities that may trigger seizures, emergency procedures

Management of Equipment

- NA

Physiological Warning Signs

- Pallor
- Irritability
- Staring
- Nystagmus
- Tonal changes
- Vomiting

Special Therapy Precautions

- Cautious use of sensory input interventions

8. Shunt

Preparation for Therapy

- Obtain history on child's signs of shunt dysfunction, emergency procedures

Management of Equipment

- NA

Physiological Warning Signs

- Lethargy
- Headache
- Vomiting
- Change in neurological status
- Bulging fontanelle

Special Therapy Precautions

- May have decreased head control, tonal abnormalities

From: "Therapeutic precautions for medically fragile infants-children," unpublished clinical tool by L.A. Geyer, 1989. Adapted by permission.

APPENDIX 4-B

Selected Neonatal Assessments

1. Neonatal Behavioral Assessment Scales (NBAS)

Publisher

Brazelton, T.B. (1973). Neonatal behavioral assessment scale. *Clinics in Developmental Medicine No. 50.* London: SIMP-Heinemann.

To Obtain Training

Required for reliability and certification; Contact Child Development Unit, Children's Hospital, 300 Longwood Ave., Boston MA 02115.

Comments

Designed for full-term healthy infants, 48 hours to 30 days old; examines the interactive capabilities of the infant; designed for research purposes, but has clinical implications.

2. Neonatal Individualized Developmental Care & Assessment Plan (NIDCAP)

Level I: Observational Training to Improve Caregiving
Level II: Assessment of Preterm Infant Behavior (APIB)

Publisher

Als, H., Lester, B., Tronick, E.Z., & Brazelton, T.B. (1982). Toward a synactive theory of development: Promise for the assessment of preterm infants' behavior (APIB). In H.E. Fitzgerald, B.M. Lester, & M.W. Yogman (Eds.), *Theory and research in behavioral pediatrics, Volume 1* (pp. 64-133). New York: Plenum Press.

To Obtain Training

Extensive training required for Level II reliability and certification; Contact Pediatric Teaching, P.O. Box 14465, Raleigh NC, 27620-4465.

Comments

The APIB designed is for research purposes, modeled after Brazelton for preterm infants.

3. Neurological Assessment—Preterm & Full-Term Newborn Infants (Dubowitz)

Publisher

Dubowitz, L., & Dubowitz, V. (1981). Neurological assessment of the preterm and full-term newborn infant. *Clinics in Developmental Medicine No. 79.* London: SIMP-Heinemann.

To Obtain Training

Directions and scoring are well described in the manual; practice and mentorship from an experienced neonatal clinician are advised.

Comments

Measures functional CNS state including neuromuscular and neurobehavioral observations.

4. Morgan Neonatal Neurobehavioral Exam (NNE)

Publisher

Morgan, A.M., Koch, V., Lee, V. & Aldag, J. (1988). Neonatal Neurobehavioral Examination: A new instrument for quantitative analysis of neonatal neurological status. *Journal of American Physical Therapy Association, 68(9),* 1352-1358.

To Obtain Training

Training workshops are available and are recommended for reliability; contact University of Illinois College of Medicine at Peoria, Department of Pediatrics, 320 East Armstrong Ave., Peoria IL, 61603.

Comments

Provides quantitative neurobehavioral assessment based on the infant's conceptual age (gestational plus chronological age).

APPENDIX 4-C

Infection Control Guidelines

Hand Washing Procedures

When to Wash

1. When coming on duty
2. When hands are obviously soiled
3. Between care of patients
4. Before and after touching one's face
5. After toilet use
6. After blowing or wiping one's nose
7. After handling materials soiled by patient secretions (e.g., dressings or diapers)
8. Before eating
9. On completion of duty

How to Wash

1. Remove jewelry from hands and wrists
2. Turn water to desired temperature
3. Apply soap
4. Rub palms together to form lather, then create friction to all surfaces of the hands and forearms for 2 minutes. Do not neglect nailbeds and between fingers
5. Rinse hands and forearms thoroughly, allowing water to flow down from forearms to fingertips
6. Dry hands completely with clean towel
7. Use unused towel to turn off water, then discard towel

Toy/Equipment Cleaning Guidelines

1. Wear gloves when cleaning toys contaminated by body fluids
2. Wipe down item with warm, soapy water, then rinse

3. Spray or wipe down with disinfectant such as 1:10 solution of 5.25% sodium hydrochlorate solution (household bleach)
4. Air dry for 10 minutes
5. Rinse well
6. Air dry

Barrier Precaution Guidelines

To Don Barrier Precaution

1. Remove jewelry, roll up long sleeves, and wash hands
2. Don gown with opening toward one's back and adjust the cuffs to fit comfortably over the wrists
3. Tie neck strings
4. Tie waist strings so that the back is fully closed, covering the clothes
5. Apply mask with metal strip facing outward and resting on the bridge of the nose. Tie top strings just over the ears
6. Pull down the lower part of the mask so that it covers mouth and chin, then tie bottom strings around the neck
7. Press metal strip over the nose
8. Apply gloves, making sure they fit snugly over cuffs of gown

While Wearing Barrier Garb

1. Be prepared to change gloves if they become torn
2. The mask is ineffective once damp; be prepared to change mask if it must be worn longer than 45 minutes

To Remove Contaminated Garb

1. Remember that all outside surfaces are considered contaminated and should not be touched with bare hands during removal
2. Remove mask and discard
3. Untie gown strings. Grasp gown at one shoulder, pull forward and off one arm. This should cause the cuff of the glove to fold over on itself. Repeat with the other sleeve
4. Remove gown, folding it so that contaminated surfaces are together and discard. Be careful not to allow your clothing to touch the contaminated surfaces of the gown or gloves
5. Use the gloved fingers of one hand to grasp the folded cuff of the other glove. Remove glove and discard
6. Now use the ungloved hand to pinch the clean surface of the cuff of the other glove. Remove glove and discard
7. Wash hands thoroughly

5

Oral-Motor and Feeding Problems

Joy Silverman McGowan, Mary Louise Kerwin, and Ken M. Bleile

INTRODUCTION

Many children receiving technological assistance experience significant feeding difficulties. Caregivers of children with **bronchopulmonary dysplasia (BPD)** commonly report difficulty with acceptance of food, vomiting and gagging, difficulty consuming adequate calories by mouth, and refusal of a variety of foods. Not surprisingly, both caregivers and health care providers typically report frustration in providing food to these children (Pridham, Martin, Sondel, & Tluczek, 1989). This chapter discusses the care of feeding disorders in children with **long-term tracheostomies** or **ventilator assistance.** The following topics are addressed:

- Oral-motor and feeding development in the 1st year of life
- Etiologic factors that cause and prolong feeding difficulties
- **Multidisciplinary** team approach in the management of feeding disorders
- Procedures for implementing a therapeutic feeding program

FEEDING/SWALLOWING

The neuroregulation of swallowing is primarily dependent on the sensation received from the pharynx and larynx and conveyed by the glossopharyngeal IX and vagus X. The cranial nerves responsible for the efferent control of swallowing are cranial nerves V, VII, IX, X, and XII (Perlman, 1991).

Traditionally, swallowing is described as occurring in three stages. In the first stage (the **oral stage**) the feeder begins to orient the mouth to the bolus. This initial stage includes the olfactory and sensory aspects of preparing for bolus reception, as well as the process of preparing and transporting the bolus. The bolus then is separated from the utensil. The tongue is shaped and goes forward and backward to move the bolus to the pharynx. While this occurs, the soft palate elevates to oppose the posterior pharyngeal wall to prevent food from going up through the nose. In the second stage (the **pharyngeal stage**) the soft palate elevates to the posterior pharyngeal wall, preventing food from entering the nose. The bolus is then moved through the pharynx. In the third stage (the **esophageal stage**) the bolus passes through the cricopharyngeal sphincter to the cervical esophagus and into the stomach.

NORMAL FEEDING AND SWALLOWING DEVELOPMENT

The anatomy of the infant's oral-pharyngeal region is designed to provide structural protection of the airway and to assist the child in acquiring nourishment. To help protect the airway, the infant's soft palate closely approximates the epiglottis, permitting food to pass directly into the esophagus. The tongue occupies most of the oral cavity, initially allowing for only front-to-back tongue movements characteristic of infant suckling. As the infant sucks, the jaw moves up and down in a rhythmic motion with the tongue. **Sucking pads,** made of fatty tissue appearing during the last month and a half in utero, provide postural stability for the infant when sucking. These sucking pads in combination with posturing in flexion allow the infant to create a suck with negative pressure.

In addition to structural anatomy, the infant possesses several reflexes that assist in feeding development. **Rooting** is a head turning reaction when the perioral region is stroked. Many newborn infants root toward the nipple when hungry or agitated. The **automatic phasic bite-release response** is an oral reflex pattern that may be elicited when tactile stimulation is provided in the mandibular gingiva or molar surface. Both the rooting and automatic phasic bite—release pattern are present at birth and gradually diminish around 3 to 4 months (Sheppard & Mysak, 1984).

At about 6 months old, the infant begins to incorporate the front-to-back movements of the tongue used in a suckle pattern with the rhythmic up and down movements of the jaw to create a munching pattern with solid foods. Over the following months and few years, the child gradually learns to use a rotary jaw movement when chewing and to manipulate the tongue to transfer food to the sides of the mouth. The youngster also learns to begin to swallow with tongue tip elevation and to use a controlled sustained bite on solid foods.

At the same time that the child's ability to feed is maturing, the natural protection of the airway decreases with the downward growth of the larynx and hyoid bone, causing a separation of the epiglottis from the larynx and soft palate. The sucking pads diminish as the oral mechanism grows.

In summary, the development of feeding consists of a series of developmental steps, each providing the infant with the ability to proceed to a more mature pattern of eating. Newborns initially use a suckle pattern to feed. The jaw moves up and down and the tongue moves in and out. Over the second half of the 1st year of life, the child gradually develops the necessary skills to manage adult foods. A more adult-like pattern of chewing and drinking emerges as the child develops more independent movements of the lips, tongue, and jaw.

IMPEDIMENTS TO FEEDING

Not all children with tracheostomies have difficulty swallowing (**dysphagia**) and feeding. There are, however, several unique experiences of the child with a tracheostomy which may impede normal feeding development. These are:

1. **Aspiration**,
2. **Gastroesophageal reflux (GER)**,
3. Reliance on tube feedings, and
4. Oral-motor experience.

Aspiration

Children with a tracheostomy seem to be prone to aspirate. Possible indicators of aspiration include a history of continuous low-grade fever or upper respiratory difficulties, "wet" voice quality during vocalization or crying and speech, coughing, and poor tongue mobility and control. In a child with heavy secretions, a "wet" vocal quality is often difficult to identify. Along with neurological deficits, aspiration is likely the result of the location of the tracheostomy tube as well as the regulation of the **mechanical ventilation** (Nash, 1988). The tracheostomy tube mechanically restricts the anterior movement of the larynx thereby contributing to the development of an abnormal swallow (Nash, 1988).

Gastroesophageal Reflux (GER)

The most common gastrointestinal problem for children with tracheostomies is GER, which is the backing up of gastric contents from the stomach into the esophagus. This is particularly likely to occur after eating. For many children with GER, eating becomes associated with nausea and vomiting.

Reliance on Tube Feedings

The nutritional needs of these children are often satisfied via tube feedings, such as **nasogastric** and **gastrostomy.** Tube feeding, especially nasogastric tube feedings, can produce negative side effects such as increased risk for aspiration (Bar-Maor & Lam, 1991), initiation or exacerbation of GER, alternation of the breathing pattern through blockage of one nostril and creating nasal and pharyngeal irritation.

Oral-Motor Experience

Experience plays an important role in the development of feeding problems. As indicated above, aspiration, GER, and tube feedings may cause the child to associate discomfort with feeding. Suctioning and tracheostomy changes may create additional aversive oral-motor experiences. Finally, feeding development can often be disrupted as a function of frequent acute illnesses resulting in periods of no oral experience.

ABNORMAL AND COMPENSATORY ORAL-MOTOR DEVELOPMENT

Aspiration, GER, and lack of experience or poor experience are capable of producing abnormal and compensatory oral-motor skills that interfere with effective oral eating. Additionally, many children with long-term tracheostomies have abnormal muscle tone and concomitant neurological deficits, which also may contribute to feeding difficulties. Motor planning problems may also contribute to abnormal oral-motor development.

The origins of abnormal and compensatory oral-motor patterns often lie early in the child's development. Low muscle tone, for example, may lead to abnormal posturing as the infant seeks to gain stability during feeding. Habitual abnormal motor movement patterns may lead to shortened musculature. To illustrate, an abnormal motor pattern may develop in a child with low muscle tone who maintains the tongue elevated to the alveolar ridge or palate to attempt to stabilize the tongue during feeding.

Another frequently observed pattern in the oral-motor development of the child with long-term tracheostomy is an inability to chew. The caregivers and/or therapists often report a child appearing to "swallow food whole." This pattern of sucking food may have resulted from the child's lack of sensory input at the posterior molar surface of the teeth throughout the sensitive period of eating development. This lack of sensory input may have led the child to avoid stimulation to the molar teeth by using abnormal compensatory movements of the tongue and lips to suck or move the food back to swallow.

There is, interestingly enough, little documentation on the impact of the tracheostomy cannula on structures and physiology of swallowing in children. It is debatable how much of a child's neck hyperextension or asymmetric head posture can be attributed to the design of the tracheostomy or is a compensatory pattern for low truncal tone. Even the high arched palate seen in most children with long-term ventilation may be related to the inactivity of the palatal muscles and not just the presence of an endotracheal tube during intubation.

ASSESSMENT

Before the assessment, the therapist should review the child's medical background to determine any existing medical issues. The clinician's review of the child's medical background includes histories of past and present upper respiratory difficulties and incidences of continuous low grade fevers. Table 5-1 lists the factors to consider when attempting to identify the children at risk for swallowing and feeding problems. Such behaviors observed frequently may indicate the need for a swallowing evaluation and appropriate medical referrals.

Before the assessment, the therapist should also note the utensils and positioning devices used during the child's feeding. The

TABLE 5-1. Behaviors indicating the need for a swallowing evaluation and appropriate medical referrals.

BEHAVIOR
Frequent episodes of gagging, coughing, choking during drinking/eating
Difficulty managing saliva (drooling)
Gurgly voice after drinking or eating
Frequent respiratory infections
Swallowing food whole
Frequent vomiting
Leakage of liquid/food from the nose or mouth
Over reaction or no reaction to liquid/food in or around the mouth
Unusual head or body movements during drinking or eating

From "Behaviors indicating the need for a swallowing evaluation" by Pennsylvania Speech-Language-Hearing Association Ad Hoc Committee on Dysphagia, 1992, *PSHA Keystater, 13*, 10.

assessment itself is performed following all the precautions described in Chapter 4 as well as any additional precautions indicated by the child's physicians and nurses.

The primary goal of the evaluation is to assess the child's feeding abilities and the status of the oral-motor system. The oral-motor evaluation should always include an assessment of the child's breathing patterns, structure and muscle tone of the oral mechanism, and presence or absence of infantile oral reflexes and drooling. Table 5-2 lists abnormal and compensatory patterns often observed in children with feeding disorders (Morris, 1982; Alexander, Boehme, & Cupps, 1993; Sheppard & Mysak, 1984; Jaffe, 1989). The feeding assessment should describe the child's ability to drink from a cup

TABLE 5-2. Abnormal and compensatory patterns often found in children with feeding disorders.

PATTERN	DESCRIPTION
Tongue thrust	Abnormal forceful protrusion of the tongue from the mouth; differs from infant suckle in range, force, and lack of rhythm
Tongue retraction	Strong pulling back of the tongue with either the tongue tip elevated or the tongue pulled back to the pharyngeal space
Lip retraction	Drawing back of the lips so that mobility is limited and lips form a tight line over the mouth
Lip pursing	Tight purse-string movement of the lips
Tonic bite reflex	Abnormally strong jaw closure when the teeth or gums are stimulated
Jaw thrust	Abnormally forceful and tense downward extension of the mandible
Jaw clenching	Abnormally tight closure of the mouth; may occur when attempting to stabilize jaw/oral musculature

or bottle and (if appropriate) proficiency at chewing solid foods and eating from a spoon. Typically, a combination of formal and informal assessment instruments are used. The procedures for these basic assessments do not differ from procedures used to assess other children with medical involvement with possible feeding difficulties (Jelm, 1990).

Specialized Assessments

Methylene Blue Screening

A **methylene blue screening** is a specialized assessment that may be performed in addition to the standard oral-motor and feeding evaluation. It is a simple procedure typically performed with children who have a tracheostomy and are potential candidates for oral feedings. The test helps to determine if the child is aspirating.

To perform a methylene blue screening, methylene blue dye or food coloring is added to the food consistency being tested. The methylene blue dye is available through a pharmacy. The child is then given food. After the child has ingested the designated amount of food, tracheal suctioning is performed and the child is monitored. If the blue dye is emitted from the tracheal **stoma** area (positive finding), then the existence of aspiration is indicated. If no blue dye appears (negative finding), then the evaluator may conclude that the food was managed without immediate aspiration. Negative findings should not be interpreted to indicate that the child is a "safe oral feeder." Negative findings only indicate that the child did not immediately aspirate that particular food at that specific feeding.

Videofluoroscopic Swallowing Function Studies

Following a complete clinical evaluation of the child's oral-motor and feeding function, the therapist may decide the child is at-risk for aspiration or that further information is needed about the child's oral-pharyngeal motility. In this situation, the therapist should review the results of the assessment with the referring physician, and together they should determine the need for a **videofluoroscopic swallowing function study.**

The videofluoroscopic swallowing function study examines oral and pharyngeal motility and determines if the child is at-risk for aspiration. The study is used to assist the staff in determining the safety of oral feeding and to provide a basis for treatment.

The study begins with the child positioned in the youngster's typical feeding posture. It is critical that the child be positioned in a posture that promotes optimal oral-motor and respiratory control.

There are many commercial adaptive positioning devices appropriate for use during the videofluoroscopic swallowing function study. The utensils, food textures, and the person feeding should be characteristic of the child's mealtime. Food textures should be presented beginning with the textures thought to place the child at least risk for aspiration.

Frank (see introductory case study, Chapter 1) provides an example of a videofluoroscopic swallowing study.

Frank

Even during the first months of life Frank demonstrated significant oral-motor dysfunction. Initially, it was difficult to determine if the feeding difficulties were related to his poor respiratory status or to his overall level of cognitive functioning.

Frank was not on a by oral (**NPO**) regimen for the first 4 months of his life because of his respiratory status and the risk of aspiration. He did not demonstrate a coordinated suck-swallow pattern on a nipple although he was able to functionally suck on a pacifier. An oral-motor stimulation program was implemented by the therapist on a daily basis. Caregiver training was inconsistent, as the mother would miss training sessions and often arrived during shift changes or in the evening hours.

By 14 months of age Frank would accept small amounts of soft food on a spoon. Thin liquids were introduced by a cup and on two occasions the nurse noted fruit juice seeping from his tracheostomy. A videofluroscopic swallowing function study was performed to obtain information on Frank's ingestion of thin liquids from a bottle and cup, thickened liquids from a cup, and puree textures from a spoon. During the study Frank was positioned upright in a custom-adapted chair. Trunk support was provided. The evaluation began with spoon feeding of baby soft applesauce mixed with barium. Three teaspoons of this texture were swallowed without difficulty. Thickened liquid was then introduced by cup and again Frank was able to manage this texture without aspiration, using a suckle-swallow pattern. When thin barium was introduced by cup, Frank coughed and began showing uncoordinated breathing and swallowing patterns. Liquids from a bottle immediately penetrated the laryngeal vestibule and a small amount was aspirated. Frank coughed and cleared the material from the laryngeal vestibule.

The recommendation of the team that performed the videofluoroscopy was to continue to spoon-feed pureed textures from a spoon and thickened liquids from a cup. It was decided that thin liquids would not be offered until oral-pharyngeal swallowing coordination improved. Bottle drinking was discontinued.

TREATMENT PROCEDURES

The major areas of therapy for children with feeding disorders are positioning for oral-motor treatment, infant suckling, stimulation of infant suckling during bottle feeding, cup drinking, reduction of fear response to solid food, spoon feeding, and chewing. Procedures to teach in each area follow. The skills need to be taught at the appropriate developmental age. Appendix 5-A lists the approximate ages at which infants acquire the major milestones in the development of feeding and swallowing. In addition, the procedures address various food types and textures. Table 5-3 defines various food types.

Positioning for Oral-Motor Treatment

Rationale

1. Facilitate optimal swallowing function.

Objects

1. Positioning or seating device such as an infant seat, chair, highchair, wheelchair, or sidelyer.
2. Materials to adapt the positioning device.

Procedures

1. Examine the child's feeding in the positioning or seating device currently used at mealtime by the family and the child's early intervention program.
2. Observe or discuss the typical mealtime environment with the child's caregiver, noting if the child is positioned at a table alone or with others.

TABLE 5-3. Definitions of food types.

TYPE	DEFINITION
Baby soft	Jarred baby food (stage 1 or 2)
Pureed	Any food blended with liquid to form smooth texture
Junior/stage 3	Pureed food with lumps and chunks
Soft textured food	Pastas, well-cooked vegetables, and so on
Textured food	Unaltered food (table foods)

3. Consult with physical and occupational therapy to determine if the seating promotes optimal body posture for feeding.
4. Determine if the child's communication system is accessible while eating.

Precautions

1. Be aware of any sign of pressure on the skin or skin breakdown.
2. Be aware of any behaviors indicating distress.

Oral Stimulation of Infant Suckling Response

Rationale

1. The infant has reached appropriate level of development in feeding.
2. The infant is a slow feeder or is unable to receive an adequate amount of liquids from a bottle to sustain health and to grow.
3. The infant requires oral stimulation exercises in preparation for eating.

Objects

1. Pacifiers of a similar shape and size to the bottle nipple being used during feedings that do not gag the child and can be easily maintained in the mouth,
2. Washcloths, gauze pads, and nonpowdered latex gloves.

Procedures

1. Schedule treatment sessions during the infant's most alert times.
2. Rub the infant's cheeks using gentle pressure in a circular motion, one cheek at a time.
3. Tap around the lips in complete circles.
4. If the infant will tolerate it, place your finger, a toothbrush, washcloth, or gauze pad in the child's mouth and massage both the upper and lower quadrants of the gums.
5. Present your finger (nail down) and rub the palate in a upward rhythmic motion (midsection to front), till suckling is initiated.
6. Stroke the midsection of the tongue in a rhythmic front to back motion.

Precautions

1. Discontinue if the infant demonstrates signs of distress or any adverse reaction (see Chapter 4 for possible signs of distress.)

Stimulation of Infant Suckling/Sucking During Bottle Feeding

Rationale

1. The infant has reached appropriate level of development in feeding.
2. The infant is a slow feeder or is unable to receive an adequate amount of liquids from a bottle to sustain health and to grow.

Objects

1. Nipples providing a steady flow of liquid to facilitate a coordinated suckle-swallow pattern.
2. Bottles that are as similar as possible to those used in the home or hospital to facilitate carryover into the child's daily environment.
3. If the child needs positioning to reduce head and neck hyperextension, use a Correcto bottle. This bottle has a nipple aligned in a position neutral to the infant's mouth with the bottle curving upward.

Procedures

1. Schedule treatment sessions during the infant's most alert and awake times.
2. Before beginning, assess for adverse reactions by giving the child a pacifier coated with formula or breast milk.
3. Introduce the bottle to the mouth using the following sequence:

   A. Stroke the nipple on side of cheek to produce a rooting response.
   B. Touch the nipple to the center of the lips and gum surfaces to help produce mouth opening.
   C. Allow the infant to close on the nipple and initiate suckling.
   D. Facilitate initiation or continued suckling using the same techniques used during oral stimulation.

Precautions

1. Medical clearance is required to begin per oral (**PO**) feeding of solid foods.
2. Discontinue if the infant demonstrates signs of distress or adverse reaction (see Chapter 4 for signs of distress.)
3. The therapist must know the signals indicating that the child may be aspirating or that the airway is compromised. These

signals are food emitting from the trachea, either when eating or later during suctioning, an increase in fevers or upper respiratory illnesses, and/or increased coughing and gagging.

Introduction to Cup Drinking

Rationale

1. Child has reached appropriate level of development in feeding.
2. Child is currently accepting only minimal amounts of nourishment from a bottle, has an absent or developmentally delayed suckle-swallow pattern, or has inadequate intake of liquids.

Objects

1. Cut-out (Nosy) cup or regular tumbler cup without the lid.
2. Thickened liquid texture (for example, thinned applesauce) that is preferred by the child.

Procedures

1. Position child in a comfortable, relaxed posture. If the child is physically impaired, position in a posture that provides the youngster the most comfort and stability.
2. Introduce the cup at other than meal or snack time in a playful situation. For example, have a doll pretend to drink from a cup.
3. Have the child place the cup to the mouth.
4. Once the child tolerates cup to their mouth, rub a preferred taste onto rim of the cup.
5. When the child accepts the taste from the cup, introduce thickened liquid from a cup.
6. When presenting the thickened liquid, rest the cup on lower lip in a neutral position in front of teeth; do not tip cup to more than a 15 to 20 degree angle.
7. Allow the child to use upper lip movement or suckle to draw the liquid from the cup. Be careful not to dump or pour liquid into the child's mouth.
8. Jaw/chin support may be provided to facilitate stability and gradated jaw movement, as well as to facilitate mouth closure and upper lip movement.

Precautions

1. Medical clearance is required to begin PO feeding of liquids.

2. The therapist must know the child's medical history, including food allergies and seizures.
3. The therapist must know the signals indicating child may be aspirating or that the airway is compromised. These signals are food emitting from the trachea either when eating or later during suctioning, congestion, an increase in fevers or upper respiratory illnesses, and/or increased coughing and gagging.

Reduction of Fear Response to Solid Food

Rationale

1. The child has reached appropriate level of development in feeding and has volitional tongue control.
2. The child needs increased caloric intake to maintain health and growth.

Objects

1. Teething toys, toothbrushes, washcloths.
2. Bagels, soft pretzels, or other firm textures that do not break into pieces and that can be easily expelled from the mouth.

Procedures

1. Schedule treatment sessions during an awake state cycle or during playtime. Do not schedule treatment sessions during mealtime.
2. Introduce nonnutritive biting experiences with smooth and soft teething toys or toothbrushes.
3. Capitalize on periods when the child is teething and more accepting of fingers and teething toys within the mouth.
4. Stimulate up and down movements of the jaw or a munching pattern by introducing food to the sides of the mouth or in between the molar surface.
5. As child gradually permits solid food to be placed inside the mouth, attempt to give the youngster more biting experience through pull and tugging games with red licorice. In these games, the therapist tugs on the licorice while the child holds tight with the teeth.
6. Potato sticks are useful in increasing the child's sensory awareness of tongue movements. Have the child hold a potato stick with the tongue elevated outside the mouth against the upper lip.

Precautions

1. The child must have volitional tongue, lip, and jaw control to expel the bolus from the mouth.
2. Medical clearance is required to begin PO feeding of solid foods.
3. The therapist must know the signals indicating child may be aspirating or that the airway is compromised. These signals are food emitting from the trachea, either when eating or later during suctioning, an increase in fevers or upper respiratory illnesses, and/or increased coughing and gagging.

Introduction to Spoon Feeding

Rationale

1. Child has reached appropriate level of development in feeding.
2. Child is currently accepting only minimal amounts of nourishment from a bottle, has an absent or developmentally delayed suckle-swallow pattern, or has inadequate intake of liquids.

Objects

1. Metal or plastic Mothercare spoon with a shallow bowl. (The Appendix of this book lists a source for custom spoons.)

Procedures

1. Position the child in an upright or slightly tilted posture. For a physically involved child, use adaptive positioning to provide comfort and stability.
2. Introduce the spoon at other than meal or snack times in a playful situation. For example, have a doll "pretend" to eat from a spoon.
3. Have the child place the spoon to the mouth.
4. Once child tolerates the spoon on their mouth, dip and coat the spoon in a preferred taste.
5. Present the spoon to the lips or front of mouth. Allow the child to actively use upper lip movements to remove food from the spoon. Do not dump the bolus of food into the child's mouth.
6. If the child's tongue protrudes, apply some pressure down on the middle of tongue with the spoon and withdraw the spoon directly out of the mouth at a neutral angle to the mouth, being careful not to scrape the spoon upward.

7. Jaw and chin support may be provided to facilitate stability, to permit gradated jaw movement, and to allow the child to use upper lip movement to close on the spoon.
8. When the child accepts the taste from the spoon, gradually increase the texture presented.

Precautions

1. Medical clearance is required to begin spoon feeding.
2. The therapist must know the child's medical history, including the youngster's food allergies and seizures.
3. The therapist must know the signals indicating child may be aspirating or that the airway is compromised. These signals are food emitting from the trachea either when eating or later during suctioning, an increase in fevers or upper respiratory illnesses, and increased coughing and gagging.

Introduction to Chewing

Rationale

1. The child has reached appropriate level of development in feeding.
2. The child currently demonstrates the prerequisite volitional oral motor movement patterns (e.g., munching) to chew and expel solid foods.

Objects

1. Solid foods varying in hardness ranging from pretzels to baby cookie textures, to scrambled egg texture.

Procedures

1. Stimulate a munching pattern in the child by presenting crunchy solid foods in between teeth (posterior molar surface). Look for up and down movement of the jaw.
2. Facilitate lateral tongue/jaw movement by stroking the lateral border of the tongue with a solid food and then placing the solid food between the teeth on the posterior molar surface.
3. While the child chews, rub the youngster's cheeks with your index finger or thumb in a circular motion, one cheek at a time to stimulate chewing or munching.
4. Jaw/chin support may be used to provide stability, facilitate gradated jaw movement, and reduce tongue protrusion.
5. As the child demonstrates increased tongue control, gradually place the food more anteriorly in the mouth.

Precautions

1. Medical clearance is required to begin PO feeding of solid foods.
2. The therapist must know the child's medical history, including the youngster's food allergies and seizures.
3. The therapist must know the signals indicating the child may be aspirating or that the airway is compromised. These signals are food emitting from the trachea, either when eating or later during suctioning, an increase in fevers or upper respiratory illnesses, and increased coughing and gagging.
4. Consistent appearance of solid pieces of food in child's stools.

Case Study

Lisa (see Chapter 1 introducing case study) provides an example of a child who was able to overcome her feeding disorder through intervention.

Lisa

Lisa's **prematurity** and the presence of the tracheostomy placed her at-risk for developing oral hypersensitivity. Lisa's caregivers were diligent in following recommendations for oral-motor stimulation activities prior to bottle feeding. They were also counseled regarding the importance of following a developmental progression in the introduction of food texture.

At 5 months of age Lisa ate pureed baby food fruits from a spoon without difficulty. She was able to suck functionally from a bottle, but was only able to take half the required calories orally. The remainder of Lisa's calories were administered through a nasogastric tube.

Unable to increase Lisa's caloric intake by bottle, the therapist introduced cup drinking at 6 months. The therapist introduced cup drinking by using a thickened liquid made of the child's preferred fruit (applesauce) mixed with apple juice. Thickened liquid was chosen to slow the oral transit of the bolus from the front of the mouth to the pharynx and to provide optimal opportunity for Lisa to use a coordinated swallow. Initially, a regular child's cup without a lid was used. The use of a regular cup facilitated the development of upper lip movements for drawing and holding the liquid in the oral cavity and providing postural jaw stability.

At 10½ months, Cheerios were introduced. Lisa demonstrated an appropriate munching pattern for solid food. These skills transferred to other solids, such as biscuits. After discharge from the hospital,

Lisa's feeding skills were monitored by her early intervention program and were found to be within the normal range in oral-motor development and ability to manage an age-appropriate diet.

A LEARNING APPROACH TO THE TREATMENT OF FEEDING PROBLEMS

For many children with long-term tracheostomy, oral stimulation and oral facilitation techniques are sufficient to produce functional oral-motor skills and patterns readily translating into eating. However, for others, these procedures and techniques are not enough. A more systematic and structured approach to treatment is often necessary.

As was discussed previously, some children may exhibit an extreme aversion toward the entire process of eating because of associated discomfort. This aversion can manifest itself in many ways—from crying when placed in the highchair to vomiting at the sight of food. These aversive reactions to the eating process make it difficult for the child to accurately and successfully practice using oral-motor skills.

Traditionally, it was thought that introducing food in a playful manner would make eating more pleasurable. Although these methods may work with some children, the techniques are typically not adequate for a child with a long-term tracheostomy. A learning approach to eating is a successful alternative. The advantages of a learning approach include an emphasis on the child's actual performance in the eating situation, the ability to use replicable methods/procedures based on systematic analysis, and the dynamic of increasing the child's success while simultaneously increasing the task demands. Through these methods, the child learns to approach rather than avoid the eating situation. (See Chapter 12 for an application of a learning approach to helping children perform self-suctioning.)

Fundamental Principles of a Learning Approach

Although it is normal for caregivers to act as teachers in other areas of a child's development, most caregivers do not think of themselves as teachers when it comes to eating. Being a teacher during feeding requires that the child be provided with feedback about appropriate and inappropriate responses, being consistent, fair, and patient.

One hallmark of effective teaching is provision of appropriate feedback by the caregiver about which responses are accurate and which are inaccurate. Infants and young children with limited language skills usually are given appropriate feedback through adult attention. When a child exhibits an accurate response, the adult usually praises the child and might even offer the youngster the opportunity to play with a favorite toy for a brief period of time. When a child does not exhibit the accurate response, the adult might not say or do anything. To help a child differentiate between the caregiver's responses (i.e., praising eating and not saying anything) as well as to maximize the child's learning capacity, a child should be fed in the least distracting environment possible until the youngster increases proficiency. The fewer the distractions, the more a child will be able to focus solely on eating.

One of the most challenging jobs for a teacher is deciding which of a child's responses are accurate. It is unrealistic to expect a child with a poor feeding history to sit down and eat a complete meal. Instead, the process of eating needs to be broken down into steps, and these steps should be within a child's capability to enhance success. For example, the appropriate first response that a teacher might expect may be a child's taking a single bite or perhaps just even sitting in the highchair with no crying.

As with adults, learning is maximized when feedback about accuracy is clear and consistent. Everyone is familiar with the confusion resulting when a supervisor says do X and the supervisor's supervisor says do Y. Adults possess the capability to request clarification; however, infants and small children usually cannot. Instead, they simply become harder to teach as they react in new ways to each different, inconsistent message. It is important for each person feeding to provide the same feedback for the same response always.

Finally, many of these children will not have eaten successfully in a long time, if ever. Setting unrealistic expectations for progress can lead to frustration. Not only will progress be slow and seemingly tedious in almost all such instances, but a person feeding can also expect that aversive behaviors (e.g., batting the spoon away) will worsen before they improve. It is extremely important that all persons feeding recognize that an escalation in negative behaviors occurs, and that consistency and persistence are the key to success. Modifying and/or discontinuing a program will only put the child again at the starting gate.

Behavioral Analysis

Because aversive behaviors can be difficult to treat, the consultation of a trained behavior analyst is essential in designing and implementing an effective feeding program for a child demonstrating food aversions. The behavior analyst will develop a comprehensive, individualized treatment for each child that should be based on (Sulzer-Azaroff & Mayer, 1991):

1. Breaking a task into small steps, with the size of each step determined by the child's ability,
2. Consideration of each step as a new opportunity for learning to occur;
3. Provision of clear instruction for the child;
4. Waiting for the desired response for each behavior;
5. Provision of appropriate consequences for each response; and
6. Gradually changing the steps as the child becomes more proficient.

Caregivers

The conceptualization of feeding as a teaching/learning experience can be very counterintuitive, confusing, and isolating to caregivers. Even some health care providers may not accept a learning approach to treatment of feeding disorders. Although caregivers may be familiar with the intensity and prolonged progress of other therapeutic programs, the response to a feeding regime appears unique.

Caregivers of children with long-term tracheostomies do not live in a vacuum. They are often faced with unsolicited and perhaps unwanted advice from friends, relatives, neighbors, and other well-wishers. Sometimes well-wishers will look askance at such an "unnatural" approach because as everyone "knows": All people like to eat. For the learning approach treatment to be successful, the caregivers must possess patience and the ability to revel in the accomplishment of small gains. It can be a very labor-intensive experience, requiring a tenacious commitment to oral feeding as a priority. Even the most committed caregivers can begin to question this approach and may even falter in their persistence, which can likely exacerbate the child's feeding problems and make future treatment even more difficult.

To persist and succeed with the learning approach, caregivers require a great deal of support and encouragement for their efforts as teachers. When advocating a counterintuitive treatment package, it is important to recognize that the health care provider is asking caregivers to place all of their trust in professional judgment. This can be very frightening for caregivers; therefore, it is important to not only offer a sound rationale for any and all feeding interventions, but to support claims with data. In addition, caregivers can be somewhat reassured when the health care provider has anticipated not only the course of treatment and the child's response in the various phases of treatment, but also the concerns of relatives and friends. Caregivers require the opportunity to discuss their concerns in a supportive relationship with health professionals.

CONCLUSIONS

The success of any feeding program depends on applicability of the program to individual patients and acceptance and agreement of the feeding plan by the caregivers, health care providers, and other adults with whom a child will interact on a consistent basis. It is essential that the feeding program be developed by a team of specialists who are familiar with normal feeding development and dysphagia. Feeding problems in children with long-term tracheostomies require oral-motor treatment activities providing children with opportunities for oral-motor sensations that the child may not customarily experience during routine feedings. Such activities provide the foundation for the development of mature feeding patterns. However, for many children with long-term tracheostomies successful oral feeding may not be attained unless the program contains a component addressing aversive reactions to food management.

REFERENCES

Alexander, R., Boehme, R., & Cupps, B. (1993). *Normal development of functional motor skills.* Tucson, AZ: Therapy Skillbuilders.

Bar-Maor, J.A., & Lam, M. (1991). Does nasogastric tube cause pulmonary aspiration in children? *Pediatrics, 87,* 113-114.

Jafee, M. (1989). Feeding at-risk infants and toddlers. *Topics in Language Disorders, 10,* 15.

Jelm, J. (1990). *Oral-motor/feeding rating scale.* Tucson, AZ: Communication Skill Builders.

Morris, S. (1982). *Pre-speech assessment scale.* Clifton, NJ: J.A. Preston.

Nash, M. (1988). Swallowing problems in the tracheotomized patient. *Otolaryngeal Clinics of North America, 21,* 701-709.

Pennsylvania Speech and Hearing Association Ad Hoc Committee on Dysphagia. (1992). Behaviors indicating the need for a swallowing evaluation. *Pennsylvania Speech-Language-Hearing Association Keystater, 13,* 10.

Perlman, A. (1991). *The neurology of swallowing.* New York: Thieme Medical Publishers.

Pridham, K.F., Martin, R., Sondel, A., & Tluczek, H. (1989). Parental issues in feeding young children with bronchopulmonary dysplasia. *Journal of Pediatric Nursing, 4,* 177-185.

Sheppard, J., & Mysak, E. (1984). Ontogeny of infantile oral reflexes and emerging chewing. *Child Development, 55,* 831-843.

Sulzer-Azaroff, B., & Mayer, G.R. (1991). *Behavior analysis for lasting change.* Chicago: Holt, Rinehart & Winston.

APPENDIX 5-A

Major Oral Motor Milestones 0-2 Years

Appropriate Amount of Food Eaten at a Meal

1 month   Takes 4 to 6 ounces of food and liquid.
3 months Takes 7 to 8 ounces of food and liquid.
5 months Takes 9 to 10 ounces of food and liquid.
7 months Takes 11 or more ounces of food and liquid.

Sucking: Liquids from the Bottle or Breast

1 month   Uses a suckling or sucking pattern with the bottle or breast. The child may lose liquid from mouth during normal sucking and swallowing movements or as the nipple is inserted or removed from the mouth.

6 months Uses a suckling or sucking pattern with the bottle or breast. The child does not lose liquid from mouth during normal sucking and swallowing movements. May continue to show a slight amount of loss at the initiation or termination of the sucking sequence as the nipple is inserted or removed.

9 months Uses a suckling or sucking pattern with the bottle or breast. The child does not lose liquid during the initiation of sucking or swallowing or during normal sucking and swallowing movements.

12 months The child no longer is given a majority of liquid intake from the bottle. Takes liquids from a cup or spoon. May continue with the bottle in the evening before going to sleep. (Note: caregiver should remove bottle before the child goes to sleep for reasons of dental care.)

110

Swallowing: Liquids

1 month   Swallows thin liquids from the bottle or breast. The tongue may protrude with an extension-retraction movement pattern during the swallow or it may simply protrude between the teeth.

6 months   Swallows liquids from the cup, with no observable elevated tongue tip position. The tongue protrudes with an extension-retraction movement pattern during the swallow or shows simple protrusion between the teeth. The lips may be open during the swallow. There may be loss of liquid from mouth.

12 months Swallows liquids from the cup with an intermittent elevated tongue tip position. This pattern may alternate with either an extension-retraction pattern or simple protrusion of the tongue between the teeth. The lips may be open during the swallow. There may be loss of liquid from mouth.

24 months Swallows from the cup with easy lip closure and no loss of liquid both during drinking and after the cup is removed from the mouth. An elevated tongue position is used intermittently to consistently for swallowing.

+24 months Swallows with no observable extension-retraction or protrusive movements of the tongue. Uses easy lip closure as needed and no liquid loss during drinking or after the cup is removed from the mouth.

Jaw Movement in Biting

5 months   Uses a primitive phasic bite and release pattern on a soft cookie. There is a relatively regular biting rhythm and lack of a sustained controlled bite through the cookie. Pieces of cookie may come off and the child may occasionally use a sucking or suckling pattern instead of an attempted bite.

9 months   Holds the soft cookie between the gums or teeth without biting through. Maintains a quiet jaw and holding posture as the feeder assists in breaking off a piece. May revert to the primitive phasic bite pattern or sucking.

12 months Uses a controlled, sustained bite on a soft cookie. When biting a hard cookie, the bite may be unsustained because of lack of teeth or biting power. The

child may revert to the primitive phasic biting pattern or sucking.

18 months   Uses a controlled, sustained bite on a hard cookie, but shows presence of overflow or associated movements in the arms or legs or head extension and pulling away to assist with the biting.

21 months   Uses a controlled, sustained bite on a hard cookie with no overflow or associated movements in the arms or legs. The head does not extend to assist in biting. When the food is presented on the side for biting, child may turn the head in the direction of the food. A full open mouth position may be used in preparation for biting food of different thicknesses.

24 months   Uses a sustained controlled bite while keeping the head in midline when food is presented on both sides. Child is able to grade the opening of the jaw appropriately when asked to bite food of different thicknesses.

From *Pre-speech assessment scale* by S. Morris, 1982, Clifton, NJ: J.A. Preston. Reprinted by permission.

6

Communication Disorders

Joy Silverman McGowan, Ken M. Bleile, Laura Fus, and Elizabeth Barnas

INTRODUCTION

This chapter describes the care of communication disorders in children with **long-term tracheostomies.** The following topics are addressed:

- Therapeutic options facilitating oral communication
- Therapeutic options facilitating nonvocal communication
- Selecting among therapy options
- Answers to questions often raised by caregivers
- Suggestions to facilitate interactions between caregivers and nonvocal infants

INTERVENTION SERVICES

Although the most direct effect of the **tracheostomy** is on phonation, the communication difficulties of children with tracheostomies typically extend beyond phonation to include disabilities in the development of both speech and language (See Chapter 1). The presence of tracheostomy in conjunction with concomitant genetic and environmental factors can serve to reduce a child's communication experiences during the first several years of life. Interactions that can be limited include babbling during the first year of life, which investigators hypothesize constitutes a type of practice activity for later speech development (Bleile, Stark, & Silverman McGowan, 1992; Locke, 1983; Locke & Pearson, 1990). Other likely missed or reduced experiences include the use of sound and words for purposes of communication, the development of verbal interactions with adults, and learning how to combine words into sentences (Bruner, 1983; Rescorla, 1989; Snow & Goldfield, 1983).

The communication development of children with tracheostomies may also be affected by hearing problems. Because of associated medical problems, many children with long-term tracheostomies are at-risk for both **sensorineural** and **conductive hearing loss,** the latter secondary to middle ear disease (Marsh & Handler, 1990). Therefore, it is extremely important that these children have periodic otoscopic examinations and audiograms (behavioral and neurophysiological) to assure that hearing is normal. Middle ear fluid problems need to be treated aggressively with medication and, if necessary, tympanostomy tubes. Sensorineural hearing loss, if detected, requires hearing aid amplification.

The goal of communication services for children with tracheostomies is to maximize the child's potential to acquire speech and language in as typical a manner as possible. In most respects children with tracheostomies receive the same assessment and therapy services as do other populations. The unique aspects of providing speech-language services to children with long-term tracheostomies are in 3 areas: (1) the medical precautions that must be observed during assessment and therapy, (2) the need to perform periodic assessments of phonation, and (3) the need to choose between the therapy options available to facilitate expressive communication. The medical precautions that must be observed when providing communication services to children with tracheostomies are described in Chapters 2, 3, and 4. The unique aspects of phonation assessment involve knowledge of a few relatively straightforward procedures. Issues involving therapy options to facilitate expressive communication are more complex.

PHONATION ASSESSMENT

Voicing by a child with a tracheostomy can only occur when sufficient air is able to leak around the cannula and pass from there up into the larynx (see Chapter 2). Speech-language therapy cannot produce voice in a child who lacks this capacity. Instead, in such a case, opportunities for phonation arise as the child grows and may allow creation of an opening between the cannula and the tracheal walls around which air can pass.

The **phonation assessment** is undertaken to determine if voicing is possible for a child and is indicated when the speech-language pathologist thinks the child has been heard phonating or a family member or health care provider reports that the child is "making sound." At the least, the speech-language pathologist should perform an assessment of phonation every 2 to 4 weeks.

The steps in the phonation assessment are:

1. Solicit the caregivers and other adults familiar with the child to determine if the child ever "makes any sounds." In considering these reports, it is important to remember that children sometimes produce sound intermittently and that caregivers may not recognize these when they occur.
2. When performing the evaluation, if possible have the child stand or sit erect. These positions keep the diaphragm from collapsing and improve the likelihood of the child being able to vocalize.
3. To elicit vocalizations, attempt to make the child excited and happy. Children tend to breathe more deeply under these conditions.
4. If unable to elicit phonation, listen when the child is crying. Typically, if a child is able to phonate, the youngster will do so at that time.

THERAPY OPTIONS FACILITATING ORAL COMMUNICATION

When selecting a mode of communication for a child, the primary goal is to provide the child with a means to express immediate wants and needs while at the same time affording the youngster a modality that will facilitate continuing speech and language development. Whenever possible, the preferred means of communication is the oral modality because, with rare exceptions (such as in the deaf culture), this is the modality of the child's family and community. Intervention options for oral communication include **speaking valves, cannula occlusion,** and **fenestrated cannulas,** which are adaptations to tracheostomies allowing air to pass over the vocal folds for vocalization; the **electrolarynx,** an electronic mechanism; and **esophageal speech** and **buccal speech,** methods relying on the use of air inhaled into the oral cavity to project sounds. For most children, the speaking valve is the therapy option of choice.

Speaking Valves

Definition

A speaking valve is a one-way valve system that fits over tracheostomy tubes with a 15 mm hub. One-way valves are used in medicine in many areas, especially in cases of pulmonary problems requiring respiratory equipment (Passy, 1986). The valves are most frequently prescribed for populations requiring tracheostomy resulting from **bronchopulmonary dysplasia (BPD),** congenital neuromuscular disorders, head trauma, and selected children receiving ventilator assistance. The principal function of a speaking valve is to allow the exhaled air to flow up the normal airway (larynx, oral, and nasal cavities). The valve achieves this effect by closing off on exhalation, forcing the air to escape through the pathway of least resistance, the normal airway.

Ward (1991) lists the following enhancements of a speaking valve on a child's communicative and overall development:

1. Overall increase in personal-social, communicative, medical, and general well being;
2. Easier and clearer vocalizations;
3. Increased air flow through the glottis, leading to increased vocal intensity, decreased breathiness, and increased sensation for vocal fold function;
4. Eliminates need for finger occlusion of the stoma;
5. Decreases oral/nasal secretions and increases expectoration (i.e., coughing, nose blowing, and so on);
6. Increases olfaction and the sense of smell and taste for oral feeds, which increases the child's appetite;
7. Helps to normalize vocal quality, intensity, pitch, and intonation;
8. Facilitates increased babbling and vocalizations;
9. Encourages increased communication and interactive play;
10. Decreases frustration;
11. Increases breath support for extended utterances; and
12. Facilitates early onset of vocalizations not usually seen in pediatric populations with tracheostomies.

Currently, there are two types of speaking valves commonly used in pediatrics. These are the Passy-Muir speaking valves and the Airlife "T" Adapter. A third speaking valve, the Montgomery, is used much less frequently. Sources for the Passy-Muir speaking valves and the Airlife "T" Adapter are listed in the book Appendix. Before recommending any valve system for a child, a medical consultation and referral is necessary. Ideally, a respiratory specialist should be present at the initial placement to monitor the child's respiratory effort while adapting to the valve. During the first few trials, the child should be monitored with a cardiorespiratory and oxygen monitor to ensure all vital signs remain stable.

The Passy-Muir speaking valves are the most commonly used and come in two styles, the tracheostomy speaking valve and the ventilator speaking valve. The Passy-Muir tracheostomy speaking valve is used with patients who do not need **mechanical ventilation** or an oxygen supply. It is designed to be closed on a bias until inspiration provides the effect of positive closure. This ensures a column of air behind the valve will protect it from occlusion. The Passy-Muir automatically closes before the end of the inspiratory cycle, with no effort required to close the valve.

The Passy-Muir ventilator valve only differs visually from the tracheostomy style in that the ventilator valve is blue and longer and is tapered to insert easily into the ventilator tubing. With the speaking valve in place, the exhalation of air passes through the trachea and out of the oral and nasal passages. The Passy-Muir ventilator speaking valve offers those children who are able to manage some breathing on their own (can breathe independently) the opportunity to speak on both inspiration and expiration, without waiting for the ventilator to cycle. Children who are unable to achieve any breathing on their own need to wait for the ventilator to cycle. The ventilator speaking valve can be adapted for patients requiring only an oxygen input line through the use of a **tracheal tube collar**.

The second device is an Airlife "T" Adapter. The Airlife is a respiratory valve that can be adapted for use as a speaking valve. Prior to adaptation, the device has both inhalation and exhalation valves. The device can be modified to convert the exhalation valve into a one-way valve (inhalation only). The valve is closed except on inhalation, which allows air to be directed through the natural pathway on exhalation. The Airlife speaking valve is designed with an open oxygen stem, allowing for connection of an oxygen input line. If the patient does not require oxygen, this open stem must be occluded with a cap to allow the one-way valve system to work. Some patients dislike the appearance of the Airlife, which is an obvious additional attachment to the tracheostomy resembling a "plastic bowtie."

Selection Criteria

1. Patient medically stable
2. Medical referral
3. Sufficient air leakage around the tracheal tube to prevent respiratory distress

Contraindications

1. Severe **subglottic stenosis**
2. Need for frequent suctioning
3. **Inflated cuff tracheal tube** or laryngectomy
4. Severe **tracheal stenosis**
5. Copious secretions
6. Unconsciousness or serious illness
7. Simultaneous use of a **humidivent** incompatible
8. Airlife "T" adapter cannot be used when the patient is on a ventilator

Therapy Procedures

Introducing a speaking valve to a child is often a challenging clinical experience. As the speaking valve affects breathing patterns, the child often requires an adjustment period before the youngster accepts the device. Some patients report that the valve creates a sensation of not allowing enough air for breathing. This sensation is caused by the additional effort needed to exhale against the resistance of the valve. Using the speaking valve also creates extra work for the respiratory muscles, as more energy must be generated to push the air around the cannula. The inability to expel secretions out of the tracheostomy may also cause distress because a child may not be familiar with coughing up secretions through the oral cavities.

To acquaint the patients with the valve, it is necessary to slowly orient them. For the first 2 or 3 days after the speaking valve is introduced (or longer, depending on the child's acceptance of the device), the child should be involved in one-on-one play with the therapist before placement of the valve. The play serves as a "warm-up" period. The child should then have the valve in place for 5 to 10 minutes during social play. The purpose of the social play is twofold: (1) to distract the child from dwelling on any strangeness in the new, alternate breathing pattern, and (2) to make the child excited, which increases the amount of energy used in breathing. This high energy state aids in the air being pushed around the tracheal tube with less discomfort. Vocal play activities when introducing the speaking valve include tickling, vocal play, laughing, and repetitions of [a]. All of the child's vocalizations should be reinforced with praise.

After the child has adjusted to the speaking valve, duration and frequency of use should be gradually increased. The exact duration and frequency of placement is determined by the caregivers and therapist based on their judgments of the patient's tolerance level. To enhance the speaking valve as a positive experience for the child, the therapist should initially remove the device before the child becomes distressed. Signs of distress include crying, irritability, and lip discoloration.

Once the child adjusts to the device and can tolerate it for 15-20 minutes, the speaking valve can be put on while the child is playing independently as well as during interactions with the therapist and caregivers. If the child is sick or has a great deal of secretions, the speaking valve may be uncomfortable and should not be worn during these periods.

Case Study

The following case study exemplifies the use of a speaking valve with a child with a tracheostomy.

Tracy was a 2-year-old socially withdrawn child who received a tracheostomy at 3 months of age because of severe BPD. She received direct oxygen input 24 hours a day and was on a ventilator at night. A speaking valve was introduced to her as a means of eliciting vocalizations. An Airlife speaking valve was chosen for her because of the need for direct oxygen input.

Approximately 2 months were required to train Tracy to tolerate the device for 10-15 minute intervals without distress. Once Tracy became tolerant of the device, intermittent 5-minute probes were conducted during play periods to assess social interactive behaviors. Data were collected when the speaking valve was in place, as well as when it was not. Outcome measures included verbalizations, prespeech oral movements (i.e., repeated labial closures, labial sputters, etc.), direct interaction with the therapist, direct interaction with a toy, and other compliant behaviors. The probe sessions were randomly alternated between valve in use and valve removed. Interobserver reliability measures were taken on 20% of the sessions, and ranged from 85% to 90%.

Table 6-1 illustrates the sum of the social communicative behaviors (vocalizations, prespeech oral movements, and direct interaction with the therapist) that Tracy exhibited during sessions with and without the speaking valve. As shown, Tracy's social communicative behaviors generally occurred at a higher frequency when the speaking valve was in place.

TABLE 6-1. Tracy's use of communicative behaviors with and without a speaking valve.

PERCENTAGE OF OCCURRENCE							SESSIONS						
100	X												
90									X				
80													X
70				X				X				X	
60			O							O			
50					X	O					O		
40							O						
30													
20		X												O
10													
0													
	1	2	3	4	5	6	7	8	9	10	11	12	13	14

X = with speaking valve
O = without speaking valve

Tracy was discharged from the hospital at 2 years, 6 months with the tracheostomy still in place. Follow-up information from Tracy's caregivers indicated that she was wearing the speaking valve approximately 7 hours a day, removing it only to eat or sleep. Her vocalizations were reported to have had greatly increased in variety and quantity. Tracy's mother reported, "We can't get her to quiet down once she has the speaking valve on." Tracy's mother also said Tracy was using her vocalizations for a variety of purposes, such as gaining attention, expressing a need for a desired object, and vocal play with toys and persons.

Cannula Occlusion

Definition

To produce voice, a leak of air must pass around the cannula to the level of the vocal folds (Simon & Silverman McGowan, 1989). However, because the air tends to follow the path of least resistance, a great deal of effort is needed to force the air past the cannula when the tracheal tube is open. Therefore, if a child with a tracheostomy wishes to speak, it is necessary to occlude the stoma to facilitate airflow through the larynx. Occlusion of the cannula is the placement of the finger, hand, or chin over the opening of the tracheal tube to temporarily occlude the cannula to block the air from exiting through the tracheostomy and, instead, pass up through the larynx.

Children who are able to produce voice through cannula occlusion are usually excellent candidates for a speaking valve.

Because finger occlusion can result in infection, the method is often most useful as a temporary means of communication or as an assessment technique to help determine if a child is ready for a speaking valve.

Selection Criteria

1. A noncritical airway
2. Not receiving ventilator assistance
3. Sufficient cognitive and language skills to understand and follow simple directions (approximately 15 months old)
4. Sufficient fine motor control to close the cannula

Contraindications

1. Lack of careful monitoring to guard respiratory status of child
2. Tight-fitting cannula (may create forced effortful vocal attempts that could result in subcutaneous emphysema)

Procedures

The goal of therapy is to train the child to occlude the cannula using either a finger or by lowering the chin. Intervention begins by desensitizing the child to having the youngster's cannula covered. This is accomplished by having the therapist slowly and playfully cover and uncover the cannula at the point when the child begins to exhale. In teaching cannula occlusion, the child should not be allowed to exhale forcibly if there is physical resistance and no sound is being produced. This is because extreme pressure could cause subcutaneous emphysema or air pockets under the skin.

After the child has been desensitized to occlusion of the cannula, the cannula should be occluded periodically during one-on-one social play situations. These situations distract the child from focusing on exhaling through the normal passageway and create high energy levels in the child that aid in pushing the air around the tracheal tube. Imitative turntaking activities can be used in which the therapist puts her finger to her neck and makes sounds, and then physically assists the child to do the same, occluding the cannula. This communication technique can be trained with relative ease when incorporated into imitative play activities.

Fenestrated Cannula

Definition

A fenestrated cannula is a tracheostomy tube with an opening within the body of the tube permitting the flow of air through the tube and across the vocal cords to allow for vocalization. Fenestrated cannulas are very rarely used with infants because (1) the plastic material of the cannula deteriorates, causing weakening of the tracheal wall, and (2) the fenestrated cannula may also place the child at risk for developing tracheal granulomas.

Selection Criterion

1. Severe subglottic stenosis preventing decannulation

Contraindications

1. Patients who are infants and young children
2. Any patient particularly susceptible to weakening of the tracheal wall
3. Frequent suctioning required

Procedures

Same procedures as for the speaking valve.

Electrolarynx

Definition

An electrolarynx is an electronic device designed to produce a vibratory sound source that can be transmitted into the vocal tract. This vibratory sound can be achieved with the electrolarynx through a mouth tube or by placement on the neck (Salmon, 1983). The device buzzes at different frequencies based on the configuration of the vocal tract. Differentiated vocal tract configurations are transmitted through the frequency of the device "buzz." Although only infrequently used with children, the electrolarynx may serve as a short-term option or a communication alternative for children not able to obtain voice through the use of a speech valve or through finger occlusion. Possible candidates for an electrolarynx include those children with aphonia from severe respiratory disease or myopathy, craniofacial anomalies, laryngeal diversion, and other neuromuscular disorders causing respiratory-phonatory incoordination.

The Servox speech aid is the most appropriate electrolarynx on the market for use with a pediatric patient. The Servox has adjustable controls for pitch and volume and an on/off switch that is relatively easy to activate. The oral connector on the Servox is not useful for a pediatric patient as the tube may become clogged with saliva and interfere with the child's articulation. The Servox is relatively expensive. (See the book Appendix for address where a price quotation can be obtained.)

Selection Criteria

1. Adequate ability to grasp and hold the electrolarynx in place and operate the on/off switch
2. Ability to perform articulatory movements without significant dysarthria or apraxia
3. Sufficient auditory skills for detection of extraneous noise from the device to adjust the position accordingly
4. Aphonia from severe respiratory disease or myopathy, craniofacial anomalies, from laryngeal diversion, and other neuromuscular disorders causing respiratory-phonatory incoordination

Contraindications

1. Inability to hold device in at least one hand
2. Inability to accommodate to loud noises

Procedures

Therapy with the electrolarynx begins with desensitizing the child to the device's noise and vibration. The child should be approached slowly, letting the youngster feel the vibration of the electrolarynx on the child's arms or legs. After this desensitization, the device might be placed on the child's face. Oral imitation activities are then conducted, with the electrolarynx near the neck. When the child is comfortable with the electrolarynx, elicitation of an audible voice is implemented.

Esophageal Speech

Definition

Esophageal speech is speech produced by swallowing air and then releasing it into the throat again. If the child meets the selection criteria to learn esophageal speech, then it is preferable to the electrolarynx as it allows the child to communicate more spontaneously. Unfortunately, approximately 40% of the patients who attempt esophageal speech fail, and, of those who succeed, acquisition of functional speech requires 6 months to 1 year.

Selection Criteria

1. The child must have a permanent tracheostomy (e.g., laryngeal diversion) or will have a tracheostomy for a very long period of time

2. Cognitive development approximates 3 years or older in order to understand procedures
3. The child does not have concomitant difficulties (such as dysarthria) that might preclude intelligible articulation
4. Good control over inspiration and expiration

Contraindications

1. Child not receiving mechanical ventilation (if the patient is ventilator-assisted, complex coordination of breathing with the ventilator is necessary, as well as injection of air into the esophagus (Simon, Fowler, & Handler, 1983)

Procedures

For inhalation, the patient opens the mouth and inhales quickly ("sniffs"), which creates negative pressure within the esophagus. This pressure differential between the esophagus and the higher atmospheric pressure in the oropharyngeal area causes air to flow into the esophagus. The patient then attempts exaggerated productions of voiceless plosives, affricates, or clusters combined with vowels (Lass, McReynolds, Northern, & Yoder, 1988).

Buccal Speech

Definition

Patients using buccal speech employ air trapped in the cheeks to produce a source of vibration. The vibrating source is then modified by the articulators to produce speech-like sound. Buccal speech is seldom sufficient for intelligible speech, but is useful to gain attention and approximate words to communicate simple requests. With continued use some children are able to speak intelligibly in 3- to 4-word sentences.

Selection Criteria

Excepting children with severe physical limitations, all youngsters with tracheostomies are potential users of buccal speech.

Contraindication

1. Some caregivers might be concerned about what might sound to them like "Donald Duck" speech

Procedures

No special procedures are needed. Buccal speech is often discovered by children when engaging in nonvocal oral-motor play. The speech-language pathologist can encourage its development through vocal play with the child.

THERAPY OPTIONS FACILITATING NON-ORAL COMMUNICATION

The oral modality may not be an option for many children with tracheostomies. These children may need to rely in part or wholly on nonoral means of communication. The principal means to augment oral communication are **manual communication** (sign language) and **alternative communication systems** (communication boards and electronic communication devices).

Manual Communication (Sign Language)

Definition

Manual communication is a nonvocal system of gestures in which the gestures are based on a meaningful symbol system (Simon & McGowan, 1989). There are two major types of sign systems: sign language, which is independent of spoken language (i.e., American Sign Language [ASL]) and sign systems, which are derived from oral language (i.e., Signed English). Sign languages are not directly related to English. In sign systems, on the other hand, signs represent English words and are produced in English word order (Davis & Hardick, 1986).

ASL is only taught to the child as a natural language in the rare situations in which the patient is the child of deaf caregivers who use that form of communication. In all other cases, the goal of teaching sign language is to teach vocabulary and to reduce the child's communicative frustration. Either the signs of Signed English or those of ASL may be used for this purpose. Employing ASL to teach such complex aspects of language as syntax and morphology is an unreasonable goal for children with long-term tracheostomies for two reasons. First, few health care workers are sufficiently fluent in sign language to use it, themselves, as a natural language. Second, even if sufficiently fluent ASL adult signers were available, the vast majority of children with tracheostomies eventually enter families and communities relying on oral communication. It is questionable whether medically ill and often cognitively compromised children should be raised bilingually, expected to acquire both sign language and oral communication.

Selection Criteria

1. The child must have a tracheostomy that will be in place during the linguistic acquisition period
2. The child emits insufficient vocalizations for purposes of communications (Simon et al., 1983)
3. Cognitive abilities minimally at the 9 month level (Simon & McGowan, 1989)
4. Sufficient motor dexterity to produce interpretable signs

Contraindications

1. Lack of adults who will potentially learn sign language
2. Severe ataxia or other motoric problems that might affect precision of signs

Procedures

With two exceptions, the procedures for teaching manual communication to children with tracheostomies are identical to procedures used to instruct other youngsters. The first exception is vocabulary selection. In addition to the typical vocabulary taught to children, children with tracheostomies should be exposed to signs referring to unique aspects of their environment. To assist the child to actively communicate its medical needs, the youngster's signed vocabulary should include concepts such as suction, tracheostomy, and ventilator.

The second exception is that, given the large number of persons likely to be involved in the child's care, it is vital for everyone to understand the signs used by the child, as well as to expose the child consistently to new signs. To facilitate the child's use of sign in a hospital, bedside diagrams should be posted detailing the signs the child knows and is being taught. Regardless of the location of care, photographs of the child performing various signs should also be posted or be readily available to help a listener understand the child's idiosyncratic signs.

Alternative Communication Systems

Definition

An alternative communication system is a system used in place of vocalizations. Examples of such systems are picture communication boards, touch talkers, and other computer systems. All types require the use of a symbol system.

Selection Criteria

1. The child must have the cognitive ability to associate symbols with meanings
2. Each individual system will have custom prerequisites for operation
3. Sufficient financial resources, if an electronic system is used
4. Insufficient patient vocalizations to permit communication

Contraindications

1. tracheostomy in-place only for short period (for electronic systems)

Procedures

There are no procedures unique to the care of children with tracheostomies. As with manual communication, the vocabulary needs to include words that permit the child to refer to the youngster's own medical needs.

CHOOSING AMONG THERAPY OPTIONS

One of the most challenging aspects of providing speech-language services to children with tracheostomies is deciding which option or combination of options best fits a given child's needs. There are at least three variables to consider when making such a decision. The first variable is the child's ability to meet the minimum cognitive, physical, and medical prerequisites to use the system. The major prerequisites are summarized in Tables 6-2 and 6-3.

The second variable is the relative advantages and disadvantages of each option as a means to reduce a child's communication frustration. Each oral therapy option reduces communication frustration because it allows the child to produce speech. Table 6-4 provides a summary of the major advantages and disadvantages of each of the major nonoral therapy options.

As indicated earlier, the first years of life are an extremely sensitive period in a child's acquisition of speech and language. An expressive communication system should provide a ladder for later development, as well as a means to meet the child's immediate needs. The third variable is the therapy benefit of a given route to the child's future communication development. All of the therapy

TABLE 6-2. Prerequisites for use of therapy options that facilitate oral communication.

COMMUNICATION OPTION	PREREQUISITES
Speaking valves	Not able to produce audible sound or vocalizes intermittently
	Medical referral
	Air leak around the tracheal tube
Fenestrated cannula	Medical approval
	Not able to produce audible sound or vocalizes intermittently
	Not infant or young child
Finger occlusion	Audible voice when crying or else vocalizes intermittently
	Helpful if child comprehends concept of stop/go
	Fine motor control to occlude the cannula is helpful for generalizing communication to various envir- onments; however, caregiver or therapist may be taught to occlude the child's cannula
Electrolarynx	Not able to produce audible sound or else vocalizes intermittently
	Child needs to be functioning at least at cognitive level of 8 to 9 months
	Sufficient fine motor control to activate on/off switch
	Sufficient auditory skills to detect extraneous noise from the device and adjust position of device accordingly
Esophageal speech	Aphonic, unable to vocalize intermittently
	Permanent or long-term tracheostomy placement (3 years or longer)
	Comprehends procedures needed to produce oro- esophageal voice (cognitive development 3 years or higher)
	Normally developing articulation skills and little or no dysarthria
Buccal speech	Agreement of caregiver

TABLE 6-3. Prerequisites for use of therapy options that facilitate nonoral communication.

COMMUNICATION OPTION	PREREQUISITES
Manual communication	Not able to produce audible sound or else vocalizes intermittently
	Sufficient fine motor control to perform signs
	Caregivers and therapists willing to learn child's sign vocabulary
Communication boards	Not able to produce audible sound or else vocalizes intermittently
	Comprehends basic objects and actions in photo- graphs or pictures

(continued)

128

TABLE 6-3. *(continued)*

Electronic communication devices	Sufficient motor control and visual focus to select a desired item on the board
	Not able to produce audible sound or else vocalizes intermittently
	Usually selected as a long-term option due to amount of technical support that is required; might be used as a short-term option if technical support is available
	Comprehends basic objects and actions depicted in symbols (words, pictures, photographs)
	Sufficient fine motor control to activate selection on a device or sufficient visual skills to operate scanning system
	Voice output desired
	Caregivers willing to learn basic operations of the device

TABLE 6-4.   Advantages and disadvantages of non-oral therapy options to reduce communication frustration.

THERAPY OPTION	ADVANTAGES	DISADVANTAGES
Manual communication	Portable Easily learned by young children (early signs are similar to common gestures)	Limited audience (not all people know sign language) Requires fine motor control to distinguish between some signs
Communication boards	Readily understood by most listeners Permits personalized vocabulary (e.g., child's own family pictures, child's medical needs)	Requires child to carry board to each environment or construction of multiple boards
Electronic communication aids	Understood by most listeners Provides audible voice for communication Permits personalized vocabulary (e.g., child's own family pictures, child's medical needs)	High maintenance (device must be charged regularly) Someone in child's home environment must have knowledge of basic programming

options provide experiences that facilitate language reception. Table 6-5 summarizes the aspects of speech development that are facilitated by each of the therapy options.

Lastly, it is important to consider how the selection of therapy options changes over time as the child grows and develops. The following examples illustrate how selection of therapy options can evolve over time. Lisa (see introductory case history in Chapter 1) provides an example of a child with a good speech outcome, whose

TABLE 6-5.   Speech experiences provided by each therapy option.

THERAPY OPTIONS	SPEECH EXPERIENCE
Speaking valves, fenestrated cannula, electrolarynx, cannula occlusion	Articulation, phonation, and respiration for speech purposes
Esophageal speech, buccal speech	Articulation and phonation
Augmentative communication	No direct speech experience, although often stimulates vocalizations while being used

communication options changed fairly quickly over a period of approximately 18 months. Another child, Mark, serves to illustrate the evolution of a child's communication system over a longer period of time.

Lisa

Lisa was entirely aphonic until 7 months, when she was given trials with a Passy-Muir valve while off the ventilator. By approximately 11 months, Lisa was able to produce reduplicated babbling when the valve was in place and was able to intermittently produce voicing even without the valve. Lisa had been exposed to sign language and by 12 months she consistently produced 5 signs. By 15 months, although Lisa continued to receive practice with the Passy-Muir speaking valve, her expressive vocabulary consisted of 7 signs and 3 oral words, /mama/ ("ma-ma"), /ba/ ("ball"), and /gi/ ("doggie").

Lisa was decannulated at 16 months. For the first several weeks after decannulation, sign language remained Lisa's primary means of communication. When Lisa spoke, her voice was soft and breathy. Over the next few months, Lisa gradually spoke more often and her use of sign language decreased. By 24 months, Lisa expressed herself almost entirely using speech. Sign language occurred for a few high frequency words (one was the name of her sister) and when Lisa was unable to make herself understood. By 28 months Lisa used speech exclusively.

Mark

Another child, Mark, provides an example of a child's changing communication needs over a longer period of time. Mark experienced much more severe lung damage than either Lisa or Frank (see introductory case history in Chapter 1) and is likely to remain tracheostomized and ventilator-assisted for his entire life. Mark was born prematurely at 30 weeks gestation and has a history of BPD, tracheomalacia, and right mainstem bronchostenosis. Mark's medical history also included cardiac arrest with an anoxic seizure in the newborn period. Cognitively, at 6 years old Mark's IQ was found to approximate 80 on the Stanford-Binet intelligence test, placing him in the low average range of intelligence.

Mark had received developmental intervention beginning in infancy and individual therapy from the time he functioned at an approximately 9-month level in cognitive development. Initial therapy goals focused on stimulating his receptive vocabulary (comprehension skills) and expanding his expressive communication skills through pointing and modeling appropriate gestures. Gestures and beginning signs were selected based on familiarity to listeners in the hospital and on the amount of fine motor ability required for the signs' production (see Chapter 4). During this period Mark indicated his wants and needs through pointing to an object or person. Because of Mark's delay in his fine motor ability, he was not always able to produce signs that persons unfamiliar with him were able to understand. For this reason, a list of Mark's signs was posted at his bedside. Photographs of Mark performing the different signs were included to help listeners better identify the signs that Mark was using.

Mark was occasionally observed attempting to imitate oral movements for speech. To provide Mark auditory feedback for his articulatory attempts, the electrolarynx was introduced during therapy. Mark was initially hesitant to use this device, but after several sessions he began to allow the therapist to position it appropriately on his neck. Carryover of the electrolarynx for his spontaneous speech attempts was not successful, perhaps because of the high turnover of staff on Mark's intensive care unit.

At 3½ years Mark was taught to synchronize his vocalization with the positive pressures he received from the ventilator. These vocalizations were intermittent and usually he was not able to vocalize more than a single one- to two-syllable word. Mark's earliest speech attempts using this method were common words beginning with consonants /m/ and /b/. Even after Mark began to use oral communication, he continued to use sign language to augment his verbal expression. Sign language was needed because Mark lacked the respiratory and phonatory control for short phrases and his articulation was often unintelligible. Mark's speech intelligibility gradually improved with time and practice. When Mark was approximately 5 years old, he was understood approximately 75% of the time by the familiar listeners in his hospital environment. Mark's use of sign language was negligible at that time.

COUNSELING OF CAREGIVERS

Counseling of caregivers and family members is a crucial role of the speech-language pathologist. Naturally, although neither the speech-language pathologist providing the counseling or the caregiver receiving the counseling is satisfied with answers such as, "I'm sorry, but there just isn't any research on that topic," it is usually the most honest and appropriate response, at present. Nonetheless, even with only the present small data base, some relatively clear answers are beginning to emerge. The questions most frequently asked by caregivers are addressed below.

Perhaps the most frequently asked question is: What will my child's speech be like after decannulation? This question is asked more frequently as decannulation approaches. Naturally, during this period the predominant caregiver emotion is one of excitement and relief that a long period of medical worries seems to be at an end. Caregivers sometimes express their relief by saying, "Now life can get back to normal." However, families also express anxiety about their child's future communication development, especially if their child had been unable to vocalize while the tracheostomy was in place. In such situations, caregivers may begin to see the child's possible communication problems as a new obstacle on the road to "getting life back to normal."

The picture emerging from recent research is that speech development is often quite slow during the months following removal of the tracheostomy, especially among children who had been unable to vocalize while the tracheostomy was in place (Bleile, Stark, & Silverman McGowan, 1992; Locke & Pearson, 1990; Simon et al., 1983). Investigators hypothesize that this slowness may result, in part, from failure to have engaged in babbling activities, which many researchers believe serves the developmental function of providing practice to the speech mechanism (Locke, 1983; Stark, 1980). For children who were unable to vocalize while cannulated, significant slowness in speech development appears to extend to at least the end of the first or second year after decannulation (Saletsky Kamen & Watson, 1991). For the reasons presented in Table 6-5, children who were able to vocalize experience quicker acquisition of speech functions after decannulation.

The slowness in speech development, fortunately, appears to be relatively short-lived. As indicated in Chapter 1, by 5 years of age language and nonverbal cognition are commensurate in virtually all children who previously had tracheostomies. Speech is delayed relative to language reception in 13% to 17% of these children. Research does not illuminate why some children have speech difficulties, and most children do not. Nor is it possible to know at this juncture if children with previous tracheostomies at 5 years old will develop speech and language difficulties as they grow older and the demands of education increase.

Another frequently asked question is: Why is a therapist teaching a child augmentative communication? In many cases, the concern (sometimes spoken, other times not) is that the therapist is "giving up on speech." The idea that their child may never speak is almost intolerable to most caregivers. For this reason, it is very important to carefully explain augmentative communication to the caregivers before it is introduced to the child. The therapist might invite the caregivers to attend or observe therapy sessions in which augmentative communication is being used to facilitate their acceptance of the therapy choice.

In discussing this therapeutic option with families, the following might be emphasized:

1. As its name suggests, augmentative communication is intended to augment speech rather than replace it.
2. Augmentative communication provides a means to reduce the child's frustration at not being able to communicate. Without some means to express needs and thoughts, the child is likely to become increasingly frustrated as the youngster grows older and wants to say more things.
3. In many cases, augmentative communication encourages speech. This may be because the child hears speech being used with augmentative communication.
4. Augmentative communication appears to encourage language development, perhaps because it allows the child a means of self-expression.
5. Before and after decannulation, augmentative communication is typically used less frequently as the child's speech abilities improve. Thus, augmentative communication appears to function as a means to help the child communicate, but does not hinder the eventual development of speech.

A frequently encountered question from caregivers of infants is: How can a therapist teach speech to a child who is too young even to communicate? Caregivers are often counseled that the therapy is "practice for speech." In many cases, the therapist may then explain that babbling and other types of sound play are thought to help children learn to practice "to get their mouths to go where they want them to go."

Lastly, many caregivers question the use of buccal speech. If this issue is raised, the therapist may counsel caregivers that buccal speech provides the child a means to communicate and that the child will cease to use it as the youngster's speech improves. If the child has a permanent tracheostomy, the caregiver may be counseled that buccal speech will not be the child's primary form of communication, as other forms will be introduced as the child develops cognitively.

SUGGESTIONS FOR FACILITATING INTERACTIONS BETWEEN CAREGIVERS AND NONVOCAL INFANTS

Caregivers often appear uncertain about how to interact with their medically involved, nonvocal infants. Because the infant is silent, caregivers may perceive the child as unresponsive. The presence of medical machinery may further inhibit caregiver attempts at interactions, as might the general unresponsiveness of an infant who is medicated or has neurological difficulties. For all the above reasons, caregivers can find interactions with their infant to be disturbing and their attempts to communicate with their child may be marked by uncertainty and hesitation.

Appendix 6-A provides a list of activities that caregivers may perform to increase interactions between them and their nonvocal infants. Caregivers should also be counseled as to why and how they should interact verbally with their infants, even though children are not able to respond vocally.

Why Verbal Interactions Help Infants

When counseling a caregiver about the need a nonvocal child has for verbal interactions, it should be emphasized that even a little infant lying in a crib is learning all the time, and that children learn about the world and how to communicate through people talking to them. Further, because the caregiver's child has been ill and in a hospital, the infant needs to be spoken to even more than other children to provide the child with the best chance to learn.

Caregivers should be reassured that, even though a child with a tracheostomy may not be able to make a sound with the mouth, the youngster still has lots of nonvocal ways to let family know what the child is feeling. Caregivers often find it comforting to be told that they'll learn to "read" their child by looking for nonvocal signs that express the youngster's thoughts and feelings, such as eye contact, eye widening, smiling or grimacing, inaudible laughing or crying, reaching, and hand-waving.

Lastly, if the infant has cognitive difficulties in addition to a tracheostomy, the caregiver might be advised to try not to get frustrated if the child doesn't seem to be learning as fast as they would like. Caregivers often need to be reminded that all children learn at their own pace, and that a child cannot learn faster than abilities allow. The value of interacting with a child is that it helps the youngster learn to that child's best ability.

Caregiver to Child Interaction

When counseling the caregivers on how to interact with a nonvocal infant, perhaps the best advice to offer is that they should talk to their child in way that is fun for the child and enjoyable and natural for them. The premise for this is that a child who has fun communicating is more likely to want to do it again.

Caregivers might be advised to keep the following questions in mind when interacting with their child: Does the youngster appear interested? Is the child paying attention? Caregivers might be advised to speak in whatever way maximizes the chance that they answer "yes" to both these questions. For most caregivers, "yes" answers are achieved most often if they use simple language when interacting with their child. Simplifying language means using short sentences and single words, talking about the "here and now," and talking about what appears to interest the child. For example, if the child appears interested in a stuffed animal, a caregiver might be advised to say, "Teddy Bear." Next, the caregiver might pet the stuffed animal, saying, "Soft," and then give the bear to the child to pet. Although such techniques are well-known among researchers in child language, some caregivers need to be reassured many times that using such simple language will not slow their child's development.

CONCLUSIONS

Communication services to children with tracheostomies are a crucial component of their (re)habilitation services. The tracheostomy has a direct impact on the ability to phonate, and the presence of the tracheostomy in conjunction with other medical and environmental factors often adversely affects the development of speech and language. The most unique aspect of providing communication services to children with tracheostomies involves facilitation of expressive communication. The principle criteria in selecting a therapy option is that it reduce the child's communic-

ative frustration and that it foster the child's continuing communication development. Selection of a communication system depends
on the child's medical status, ability to pass air around the
tracheostomy tube, and other physical necessities.

Oral techniques include speaking valves, cannula occlusion,
fenestrated cannula, electrolarynx, esophageal speech, and buccal
speech. Other nonoral techniques include manual communication
and alternative communication systems. For most children, the
speaking valve is the therapy option of choice. Regardless of the
system chosen to facilitate communication while cannulated, it is
necessary to be prepared to counsel the caregivers and family members regarding the child's current and future communication
abilities. Additionally, many caregivers of nonvocal infants require
assistance in understanding why and how to interact with their
child.

REFERENCES

Bleile, K., Stark, R., & Silverman McGowan, J. (1992). *Evidence for the relationship between babbling and later speech development.* International Symposium on Clinical Linguistics and Phonetics. London, England.

Bruner, J. (1983). *Children's talk: Learning to use language.* New York: Norton.

Davis, J., & Hardick, E. (1986). *Rehabilitative audiology for children and adults.* New York: Macmillan.

Fowler, S., Simon B., & Handler, S. (1983). Communication development in young children with long-term tracheostomies: a preliminary report. *International Journal of Otorhinolaryngology, 6,* 7-50.

Lass, N., McReynolds, L., Northern, J., & Yoder, D. (1988). *Handbook of speech-language pathology and audiology.* Toronto: B.C. Decker.

Locke, J. (1983). *Phonological acquisition and change.* New York: Academic Press.

Locke, J., & Pearson, D., (1990). Linguistic significance of babbling: Evidence from a tracheostomized infant. *Journal of Child Language, 17,* 1-16.

Marsh, R., & Handler, S. (1990). Hearing impairment in ventilator dependent infants and children. *International Journal of Pediatric Otorhinolaryngology, 20,* 213-217.

Passy, V. (1986). Passy-Muir tracheostomy speaking valve. *Otolaryngology: Head and Neck Surgery, 95,* 247.

Rescorla, L. (1989). The language development survey: A screening tool for delayed language in toddlers. *Journal of Speech and Hearing Disorders, 54,* 587-599.

Saletsky Kamen, R., & Watson, B. (1991). Effects of long-term tracheostomy on spectral characteristics of vowel production. *Journal of Speech and Hearing Research, 34,* 1057-1065.

Salmon, S. (1983). Artificial larynx speech: A visible means of alaryngeal communication. In Y. Edels (Ed.), *Laryngectomy: Diagnosis to rehabilitation.* London: Croom Helm.

Simon, B., Fowler, S., & Handler, S. (1983). Communication development in young children with long-term tracheostomies: Preliminary report. *International Journal of Pediatric Otorhinolaryngology, 6,* 37-50.

Simon, B., & Silverman McGowan, J. (1989). Tracheotomy in young children: Implications for assessment and treatment of communication and feeding disorders. *Infants and Young Children, 1,* 1-9.

Snow, C., & Goldfield, B. (1983). Turn the page please: Situation-specific language acquisition. *Journal of Child Language, 10,* 551-569.

Stark, R. (1980). Stages of speech development in the first year of life. In G. Yeni-Komshian, J. Kavanagh, & C. Ferguson (Eds.), *Child phonology: Production.* New York: Academic Press.

Ward, P. (1991, November). *Use of the Passy-Muir valve in the pediatric tracheostomized population.* Paper presented at the annual meeting of the American Speech-Language-Hearing Association, Atlanta.

APPENDIX 6-A

Interaction Activities for Caregivers With a Nonvocal Infant

If caregivers appear to have difficulty in interacting with their nonvocal infant, the following advice might be of assistance.

1. Good times to talk to your child are while playing together and in performance of such daily activities as bath time, diaper changing time, and mealtime.
2. Greet your child when you first see the youngster and say good-bye when you leave. Look for eye contact and smiling as signs that your child is aware of you. If your child doesn't appear to be paying attention, sit face-to-face when greeting your baby and saying good-bye.
3. Most infants like to play with rattles. To start with, shake the rattle on the left side and then the right side of your child. Later, let your child hold and shake the rattle. Watch for eye widening, head turning, and body movements as signs that your child is interested and enjoying the activity.
4. Play tickling games. Starting when your child's development is about that of a 5-month-old infant, creep fingers toward her, saying something like, "Here come my fingers. Here they come to get you." Signs that your child is enjoying this game include inaudible laughing and body movements.
5. Beginning when your child's development is about that of an infant 7 months old, begin to mirror play with your baby. Position your child for self-viewing in the mirror. Say something like, "That's _____ Who's that? It's _____" Allow your child to touch the baby's mirror image. Look for signs of smiling and puzzlement.

6. Play peek-a-boo games. Starting when your child's development approximates that of a child 5 months old, cover your child's head with a little blanket, being careful of the tracheostomy tube. Ask, "Where's _____?" Then lift the blanket, saying, "There's _____!" As your child grows, play peek-a-boo covering your eyes with your hands, asking, "Where's _____?" Then put your hands away from your eyes, saying, "Here's _____!" Clap, and then say, "Now it's your turn." Help your child put hands over eyes for the baby's turn, if requiring assistance. Speak the words that are part of the game for your child. Lastly, peek-a-boo can also be played with objects. Place a small blanket over an object such as a doll or toy, and ask, "Where's the _____?" Let your child uncover the object or touch the object for you to uncover. Alternately, you can slowly pull the blanket off the object, exclaiming, "There it is!" Signs that your child is enjoying these games may include smiling, inaudible laughing, and movement of arms and legs.

7

Developmental and Behavioral Issues

Jean L. Fridy and Kathleen Lemanek

INTRODUCTION

Developmental and behavioral issues associated with **long-term tracheostomy** and **ventilator assistance** are receiving more attention as the number of children aided by these technologies increases. As a child's survival becomes more certain, caregivers and health care providers face the challenge of optimizing quality of life in terms of enhancing cognitive function, social competence, and emotional adjustment.

In this chapter, developmental and behavioral issues as relating to long-term tracheostomy and mechanical ventilation are discussed. The chapter focuses on providing psychological services to children who undergo frequent and lengthy hospitalizations. The reason for focusing on this population is that the combination of hospitalizations in conjunction with technological assistance required to maintain the airway presents a particular challenge in providing psychological services to the child, caregivers, and the professional members of the health care team. The following topics are addressed:

- The nature of the developmental and behavioral issues arising in the care of children with long-term tracheostomies
- Assessment of cognition and behavior
- Treatment of cognitive and behavioral disorders

• The psychologist's role with caregivers and other members of the health care team

DEVELOPMENT

Cognitive Development

Studies of the developmental status of children supported by tracheostomies and ventilators for lengthy periods are scarce (see Bleile, this volume, for a review of the outcome studies). The existing studies are limited in generalizability because of small sample sizes, heterogeneity of subjects, variability in medical care, and gross assessment measures. Even with this caveat, the findings are sobering, especially for children receiving mechanical ventilation.

There are, nonetheless, many factors affecting development that are modifiable. Although children with long-term tracheostomies or receiving ventilator-assistance are medically fragile and at high-risk for developmental disabilities, the relationship between a child's biology and the youngster's environment is a transactional one, and each may either limit or counteract the other (Lerner, 1987). Sameroff and his colleagues (Sameroff, 1981; Sameroff & Chandler, 1975) find that a child's social environment is a better predictor of outcome than **perinatal** factors. It appears that within certain parameters, such as when neurophysiological status is not severely compromised, a healthy, stimulating environment can counteract the effects of early physical trauma. Conversely, impoverished environments can exacerbate organismic vulnerability.

The case of Frank exemplifies such a situation (see introductory case history in Chapter 1); his family's inconsistent attendance at training sessions and reluctance to accept his initial discharge date resulted in his spending an additional 4 months in the hospital. At 48 months he was functioning in the moderate range of mental retardation with moderate to severe behavior problems. His mother's drug use during pregnancy and continued use after his return home interfered with her ability to provide a consistent, stimulating environment. Although it is unlikely that Frank's level of functioning would have risen to a normal range in a different environment, the possibility does exist that his cognitive skills could have developed better, and more likely, his behavior be less problematic. In contrast, the case of Lisa (see introductory case study, Chapter 1) shows the steady developmental gains of a child supported by multiple and extensive therapies and a strong, nurturing family.

One must ask then: Given a child's medical needs, what aspects of the hospital environment interfere with growth and development and can these elements be modified? Many children who are tracheostomized or ventilator-assisted do not have severe neurological damage. For these children, the environment may have more impact, either exacerbating biological vulnerabilities or counteracting them.

Environmental Effects

The early research investigating the effects of institutionalization on young children's cognitive development was discouraging (Spitz, 1945). Those early studies find serious developmental handicaps associated with long-term care; later research in nurturing orphanages where children received considerable individualized attention from staff suggests that, although children emerge from such experiences with developmental delays, they can recover substantially if placed in healthy home environments (Tizard & Hodges, 1978; Tizard & Rees, 1975). Although the hospital setting of today is a far cry from the mostly sterile institutional environments of the past, any facility retains some of the negative features of an institutional setting. Multiple caretakers, staff turnover, routinized care, and aversive medical procedures, in combination with the lights and noise of the hospital unit, contribute to an environment that is insensitive to individual needs, unpredictable, and overstimulating (Thoman, 1987). Moreover, the scarcity of toys, limited opportunities for pleasurable physical contact, and physical confinement make hospitals understimulating environments, as well.

Most of the children hospitalized for chronic respiratory failure are under 2 years of age and in the sensorimotor stage of development. For these children, limited physical mobility impedes the exploration and interaction with the environment crucial to the attainment of the developmental tasks of the sensorimotor period, such as awareness of self and objects in space, cause and effect, and object permanence. Constant adult supervision outside of the crib and extended periods unattended in the crib deny the hospitalized child the opportunity to "cruise" the area, engage in the repetitive but satisfying acts of dumping and filling and rearranging available to infants and toddlers at home. The hospital unit does not have closets full of shoes and inviting trash cans available for the young child to investigate. Although everyone is well aware that children should have access to a variety of toys and objects (Yarrow, Rubenstein, & Pedersen, 1975), to provide such opportunities to children whose respiration must be monitored, lungs cleared, tracheostomy tubes changed, and blood levels drawn requires a major commitment from nursing and support staff. Moreover, the everyday experiences of the hospitalized child are unique to the hospital culture, obscuring and occasionally substituting for the child's own cultural customs and norms. The child on a specialized ventilator unit does not feel wind on the face, hear the sound of traffic, walk in the park, nuzzle a puppy, or see meals prepared.

Development of Relationship

The infant hospitalized for an extended period of time, particularly one supported by a ventilator, is at a tremendous disadvantage for psychosocial development. Not only does the child's limited mobility interfere with a sense of mastery and competence, but the presence of multiple caretakers and the uncertain role of the caregiver interferes with the development of personal relationships. Given that the developmental task of the infant is to establish a sense of trust (Erickson, 1963), presumably through the development of a secure attachment relationship, the hospitalized infant must overcome a plethora of obstacles to accomplish social goals.

The customary avenues to eliciting caretaking behaviors from attending adults, such as sucking, crying, smiling, clinging, and following, are often compromised. Bowlby, in his seminal work on attachment and separation (1960, 1961) describes these behaviors as genetically based signaling devices intended to cue the caretaker to the infant's needs. Whereas the healthy infant is viewed as an active contributor to the development of an attachment bond (Bell & Ainsworth, 1972; Stern, 1974), the medically ill child is significantly less effective in influencing the caretakers' behavior. To illustrate, the child is often tube-fed, thereby denied the physical and visual interaction that accompanies the traditional, pleasurable, feeding routine. Normally, the infant sucks, stops, and looks at the feeder, who then may smile, talk to the baby, stroke or jiggle the infant. The baby's hunger is satiated in a highly charged social and emotional context. The child who is tube-fed for months is denied that pleasurable exchange, may experience feeding problems later (see Chapter 5) and, more importantly, is handicapped in efforts to develop satisfying personal relationships.

Perhaps the most striking (and poignant) feature of a hospital unit devoted to the care of children with tracheostomies is the silence. Alarms and adult voices prevail. Children are unable to produce the cries that signal distress and reliably provoke adults' caregiving responses. A silent crying infant may go unnoticed by busy staff, and a baby who is noticed, is more easily ignored. A busy adult who moves out of sight of a silently crying infant may forget the child in distress without the ongoing and compelling reminder of a full-blown cry. Lacking perhaps the most powerful signaling behavior, the infant must find other ways to communicate needs.

Individuation

Normally, the toddler crawls or walks away from an adult, using the grownup as a secure base from which to explore (Ainsworth & Bowlby, 1991). The child will regulate the timing and the distance of brief separations, using visual and vocal modalities to maintain contact. This leaving and returning allows the child self-experience as an individual, separate from others. The process of individuation continues throughout the lifespan. The child whose mobility is limited by technology is handicapped in efforts to develop this more mature attachment bond, a sense of self as a separate person, and a sense of mastery in relation to an individual's environment. Independence, the principal psychosocial goal of the toddler (Erickson, 1963), is difficult to obtain. Attached to a tracheostomy tube and ventilator and often confined to a crib, the toddler is unable to cling to or follow the youngster's caretaker. The hospitalized child does not experience the control the mobile toddler wields over a relationship with a caregiver.

Reciprocity

Caregivers foster healthy attachments by sensitive and consistent responsiveness to their children's needs (Ainsworth & Bowlby, 1991). However, caregivers of children assisted by technology may be confronted with numerous obstacles with the potential to interfere with their ability to bond with their child. Ambivalent feelings toward the child, distance from the hospital, job and family responsibilities may be overwhelming. A highly committed caregiver still may find the child's cues difficult to read and might experience the child as unresponsive (see Chapter 6); the caregiver may be intimidated by the technology surrounding the child or by the competence and assurance of the medical staff. Young, first-time caregivers, particularly those with limited resources, find it particularly difficult to remain actively involved for months or years at a time under these circumstances. Frank's family responded to this stress by delaying his discharge.

Mastery

Children who establish a healthy relationship with a caretaker experience the accomplishment of influencing the behavior of another human being. Over time, the child develops a sense of competence and mastery over the youngster's own environment. However, the caretaking behaviors of staff and caregivers are often noncontingent on the behavior of a hospitalized child assisted by technology. The child may be fed on a schedule or held only when time is open; procedures may need to be performed regardless of the child's protest. The characteristics of reciprocity and the fine tuning in successful and secure attachment relationships are limited. The child's experiences of effectance are restricted, increasing the likelihood not only of attachment delay and/or disruption, but also the behavioral passivity characteristic of the "learned helplessness" described by Seligman (1975). The child may turn to maladaptive means to secure adult attention, such as disconnecting leads or retreat to self-stimulation. Setting off alarms is highly reinforcing; it produces a predictable adult response and secures attention. Self-stimulating behaviors are reinforcing as well, but serve to further isolate the child from the environment. And, efforts at discipline in a hospital will often be inconsistent, coming from a variety of sources and not usually as effective as when discipline sources are emotionally important to the child (Ainsworth, Bell, & Stayton, 1974; Ainsworth & Bowlby, 1991).

Socialization

Lastly, the social interactions and adaptive functioning of young children growing up in a hospital setting can be restricted. Playmates are often limited to other children on ventilators and spontaneous opportunities for play and socialization are infrequent. Curtains may be drawn, a child's mobility may be variable, and time is filled by treatment needs. Often, interactions with many people are superficial, restricted by sheer numbers, turnover, and other job responsibilities. Children do not participate in the normative cultural routines, such as a social meal time, dressing, cooking, and toileting and bathing in the bathroom. Not only are children "culturally deprived" (though they do certainly absorb the hospital culture, and may be well versed in medical procedures), they are seldom encouraged to assume responsibilities for themselves. It is easier for staff to dress, bathe, and diaper young children than to teach them to care for themselves. This may not be an issue for children such as Frank and Lisa, hospitalized for comparatively shorter periods of time, but it is for children who may spend years in rehabilitation hospitals.

Behavior

Deviant behaviors that may be characterized as attention-seeking (e.g., disconnecting tubing from the ventilator thereby sounding the alarm) or aggressive (e.g., scratching staff), and episodes of self-stimulation (e.g., body rocking) and/or self-injury (e.g., **decannulation**) may occur among children with tracheostomies. The literature indicates that such behaviors are common in children who are functioning in the mentally retarded range of development, a characteristic of many children who are technology-assisted and on a rehabilitation unit. However, the extent to which these behaviors are attributable to organismic variables, environmental variables, or a combination of both needs to be determined for each child individually.

Operant Conditioning

Three hypotheses, based on **operant conditioning theory**, have provided a conceptual framework for the study of variables functionally related to self-injurious behaviors (Carr, 1977). These hypotheses may be applicable to research on the aberrant behaviors of children who are technology-assisted.

The first hypothesis proposes that the development and maintenance of aberrant behaviors may be a function of **positive reinforcement** in the form of attention received by others (Mace, Lalli, & Shea, 1992). Attention can vary greatly from, for example, a mild disapproving look to a loud reprimand, or from a look of sympathetic concern to a physical embrace and expression of sorrowful consolation (Mace et al., 1992). The second hypothesis suggests that **negative reinforcement** maintains these behaviors when the behavior results in escape or avoidance of certain situations or demands. The final hypothesis states that aberrant behaviors may be maintained by the sensory stimulation produced by the behavior itself. The degree to which these hypotheses fit the conceptualization of aberrant behaviors in children who are technology-assisted requires empirical investigation, which should be a priority of future research.

Classical Conditioning

A paradigm based on **classic conditioning theory** may also be pertinent to the conditioning of aberrant behaviors in these children: conditioned suppression. Research on conditioned suppression has shown that in situations where there is strong, unpredictable, unavoidable, and escapable aversive stimulation possible reactions are: (A) suppression of appetitive and goal-directed behaviors, (B) stopping of defense behavior (avoidance and escape responses) if aversive stimulation continues, and (C) biological responses (e.g., changes in gastric secretions and brain amines) (Cataldo, Jacobs, & Rogers, 1982).

Cataldo, Bessman, Parker, Pearson, and Rogers (1979) conducted one of the few empirical studies on the behavior of children in an intensive care unit (ICU); their findings are striking and related to the conditioned suppression paradigm. In this study, observations and analysis of children's state, physical position, affect, verbal behaviors, visual attention and activity engagement, and staff verbal behavior were conducted. Results reveal a general lack of behavior in terms of minimal verbalizations and engagement in activities. For example, most of the time the children were not engaged in any play activity; they were most often scanning the environment or staring into space. Those who were engaged usually played in the presence of another person, but not when alone. In addition, the affect of the children was not negative but neutral 58% of the time when awake. Again, it is unclear to what extent these results can be generalized to other children, such as those who are technology-assisted and on a rehabilitation unit for an extended period of time.

COGNITIVE ASSESSMENT OF THE CHILD WHO IS HOSPITALIZED

Assessment Areas

The skill areas that should be assessed in children who are technology-assisted are not substantially different from those examined in children with other medical conditions or evidencing developmental delays. Clearly, the array of factors affecting these children's development renders a formal assessment protocol unrealistic. However, to obtain a representative sample of the child's skills in different areas the assessment should be comprehensive, including an estimate of overall cognitive development, play, adaptive behaviors, receptive and expressive language skills, nonverbal skills such as visual discrimination and imitation, and visual and auditory memory skills. These areas should be assessed at varying stages to document strengths and weaknesses and to monitor skill development or deterioration during the hospitalization.

Method

The assessment methods used with children who are technology-assisted are more similar to than different from those utilized with other children. However, the specific procedures and the timing of the assessment may differ to varying degrees, depending on both medical and developmental variables. In this respect, several issues need to be considered and questions asked before beginning the assessment.

Medical Considerations

Relevant medical information is necessary to interpret results of any evaluation. Examples of the most critical information to review include the child's medical diagnosis, gestational history, reason for the ventilation and length of time required to be on mechanical support, other medical conditions or complications (e.g., scoliosis, nasogastric tube feedings as sole means of nutrition or as supplements), documentation of neurological insults, and recent changes in the child's respiratory condition or oxygen requirement. The latter issue relates to a possible association between increased irritability and decreased activity level, along with reduced in breaths per minutes and/or extended time off the ventilator.

A second but related issue is determining if the child is on any type of medication that might negatively affect behavior or performance during the evaluation; for example, increased irritability has been identified with administration of phenobarbital.

A third issue is elimination of to what degree, if any, the equipment (e.g., ventilator and feeding tubing) interferes with the child's exploratory behaviors, play activities, and social interactions with adults and other children; the development of a child's sensorimotor schemata may be adversely influenced if such activities are limited.

Fourth, any equipment influence on administration of the tests requires examination. For example, these children almost always need to be evaluated in cribs or high chairs located in their rooms, with all the varied and, for the most part, uncontrollable distracting stimuli of a hospital unit. Finally, the most "workable" time for conducting the assessment needs to be explored, especially with the nursing staff, to schedule best in line with the child's routine care schedule, program of medical treatments, and availability of staff to participate in the assessment session.

Standardized Assessment

An ample number of standardized tests are available to assess the general cognitive abilities and specific developmental skills of children who are technology-assisted, each tool having its own psychometric strengths and weaknesses. The specific test(s) chosen should depend on the purpose for which the assessment is to be used: whether screening of general cognitive development, formal evaluation for diagnosis and/or classification, or assistance in placement decisions and/or treatment recommendations.

The specialized tests most often administered include the *Bayley Scales of Infant Development* (Bayley, 1969), *Gesell Developmental Schedule* (Ilg & Ames, 1965), and the *Extended Merrill-Palmer Scale* (Ball, Merrifield, & Stott, 1978), because many, if not most, of the children admitted to a rehabilitation unit are below the age of 2 or evidence significant delays in multiple skill areas. When a child's skill development is beyond the age of 2, one of the more psychometrically sound standardized tests of intelligence should be administered, such as the *Stanford-Binet Intelligence Scale—Fourth Edition* (Thorndike, Hagen, & Sattler, 1986) or the *Wechsler Primary and Preschool Scale of Intelligence—Revised* (Wechsler, 1989). Administration procedures for portions of these tests might need to be modified to accommodate the special requirements of the target population. However, when making those adaptations, one must continue to acknowledge the deviation from standardized administration procedures in careful evaluation of findings. Detailed information about test features, administration, and psychometric characteristics of these measures can be found in Sattler (1988).

In terms of play skills, the *Symbolic Play Test* (Lowe & Costello, 1976) has been used with children who are technology-assisted. Informal evaluation of play skills can be conducted within either unstructured or structured situations in the child's room and/or play room of the hospital. Toy play can be observed and recorded according to the level of play engaged in by the child: manipulative, relational, functional, and symbolic based on the work of Piaget (1967) and others (e.g., Lowe, 1975).

BEHAVIORAL ASSESSMENT OF THE HOSPITALIZED CHILD

Content

Assessment of responses of children who are technology-assisted should not only focus on aberrant behaviors, but also on prosocial or adaptive behaviors. What skills are in the child's repertoire to elicit attention from staff, therapists, and other caregivers? Does the child respond to social interactions by smiling and/or laughing? To what degree can the child assist in self-care or demonstrate adaptive behaviors (e.g., dressing, self-feeding)? How well does the child engage in both independent and assisted play activities? Answers to these questions, as well as others of this type, will provide information on the level of adaptive behaviors within the child's inventory.

Methods

A multimethod approach in the assessment of behaviors of children who are technology-assisted is essential for accurate and useful information to be integrated for both understanding and remediating behavioral concerns (Mash & Terdal, 1981; Ollendick & Hersen, 1984). Numerous assessment strategies are available to obtain this information, although such methods as the clinical interview and behavioral observation may be the most fruitful to employ. In any event, the assessment strategies utilized must be sensitive to developmental changes in a given child, both expected and unexpected, from "normal" processes or medical complications (Mash & Terdal, 1981; Ollendick & Hersen, 1984). Finally, the child's behavior should be assessed within an ecobehavioral framework (see Bronfenbrenner, 1979), in which the behavior and its controlling variables are analyzed at the individual level, the microsystem level (e.g., hospital room), the exosystem level (e.g., rehabilitation unit), and the macrosystem level (e.g., hospital).

Clinical Interview

There exists a wealth of material on the definition, goals, reliability and validity, and guidelines for conducting an effective clinical interview (e.g., Haynes & Jensen, 1979; Linehan, 1977). The goals of a clinical interview are to gather information about the referral concerns and aims, acquire relevant historical data, and identify environmental and organismic variables serving to maintain problematic behaviors, including antecedents and consequences (Haynes & Wilson, 1979). It is critical to obtain a precise description of the problematic behaviors and the situational variables related to the conduct, because of the relationship with other methods of assessment (e.g., designing a behavioral observation system) and to treatment strategies (e.g., selecting target behaviors) (Ollendick & Hersen, 1984). When conducting interviews in a hospital setting, greatest attention should be given to collecting information on organismic variables relevant in other settings; organismic variables can include individual differences produced by remote environmental influences (e.g., past learning in the pediatric ICU), genetic factors (e.g., fragile X syndrome), and current physiology (e.g., hunger, fatigue) (Kanfer & Saslow, 1969).

The sources of information for an interview can be quite varied in a hospital setting. The most valuable sources include the child's primary nurse, one or two nurses who regularly care for the child during the day and the evening shifts, other relevant therapists who work with the child in different situations (e.g., physical therapy, recreational therapy), and, if possible, family members. As they will probably be the staff implementing treatment protocols on the unit, it is extremely important to determine during interviews how receptive the nursing staff or other therapists are to different types of treatment strategies (e.g., time-out versus ignoring).

Naturalistic Observations

Observation of behavior in the "natural environment" is considered the hallmark of behavioral assessment (e.g., Foster & Cone, 1980; Nelson & Hayes, 1979). In general, conducting a systematic behavioral observation on a rehabilitation unit, or elsewhere in a hospital, is extremely difficult. It is time-consuming for both the staff and the person collecting the data as well as compounded by numerous variables related to administration of treatments and therapies (e.g., observers need to be trained to record behavior based on strict operational definitions of the behavior). In fact, behavioral observation is an assessment strategy used less often in clinical practice than in research because of the paucity of available standardized observational instruments (Jones, Reid, & Patterson, 1975) thereby dictating development of one's own system that may or may not be adequate or psychometrically sound. Through whatever means behavioral observations are conducted, obtaining a representative sample of the target behaviors is mandatory. That is, observations need to be made of the child across settings (e.g., room, playroom on unit, off unit), across situations within settings (e.g., during medical procedures, when alone, in group versus solitary activities), and across time (e.g., different days and shifts).

An alternative strategy to behavioral observation is for staff and/ or family members to monitor, in a systematic manner, the behaviors of interest. The method of recording the child's behavior needs to be easy to implement but also result in a representative sample of the child's behavior, as in behavioral observations. Frequency counts, time-sampling procedures, spot checking, or outcome measures (e.g., change in body weight) are examples of methods of recording (Haynes & Wilson, 1979). Monitoring by others of the child's behavior appears to be generally the most feasible method of assessment as recording times and method can be assimilated and accommodated into the staff's routine.

INTERVENTION WITH THE CHILD IN A HOSPITAL

The complex medical, developmental, and social needs of children who are technology-assisted demand the design and implementation of a comprehensive treatment program. Frequently the foci of treatment are on the iatrogenic effects of necessary but invasive medical care and the functional impairments stemming from the medical conditions. However, intervention to habilitate cognitive and/or behavioral impairments should be directed not only toward individual children but also toward the environment. The thoughtful design of patient rooms and entire units can prevent or limit the scope of problems.

Cognitive

Preventive Measures

Premature birth and its complications, such as respiratory difficulties, are a source of central nervous system (CNS) insult for infants (Bendell Estroff, in press). Although little is known about the optimal conditions for promoting the cognitive and emotional development of these infants (Bendell Estroff, in press), there are virtually no data on children who are technology-assisted. However, one can generalize from the literature on the intensive care experience of premature infants to children assisted by technology. For example, the provision of an optimal level of social and physical stimulation has been reported to soften the impact of an early neurological injury (Gorski, 1983). Furthermore, premature infants are considered less able to block out intrusive stimuli and, therefore, need environmental protection from such aversive stimulation (Bendell Estroff, in press).

Until data are disseminated indicating at what point infants and children do not need such environmental support, rehabilitation rooms and units should be environmentally designed to resemble intensive care units. For example, dimming the lights on a regular schedule, reducing talk across beds and rooms, and moving television sets out of the rooms and into the commons area of the unit are simple and effective strategies. Other strategies that may be more applicable to a rehabilitation unit with children who are technology-assisted include drawing curtains around the crib/bed during medical procedures or performing as many medical procedures as possible off the crib/bed (e.g., suctioning), setting up specific areas of the unit where children can eat meals together (or at least be a part of the "family" if tube fed) rather than eat in their rooms in high chairs, and obtaining portable ventilators so children can ambulate in the middle of the unit at scheduled times and/or go to different parts of the hospital with only minimal inconvenience.

Direct intervention

In addition to these environmental changes, development of an adequate stimulation program for each child is mandatory. One method of providing services is to integrate any early intervention program sponsored by an area public school system into the hospital setting. Development of intelligence during the first 18 months of life is reportedly dependent on the child's ability to move and to explore the environment (Dalton & Kirkhart, 1985). The mobility of children with tracheostomies who are also ventilator-assisted is restricted by limitations imposed by equipment as well as by the hospital unit (e.g., decreased opportunities to ambulate). It is critical that these children be provided the means to learn about and to explore their environment.

Numerous strategies can be incorporated into the child's treatment program to develop and shape play, exploration, and attention. For example, the play area should be structured with toys organized and accessible (not haphazardly placed in the room or crib/bed), a series of toys rotated every few days, manipulation of the toys described, and adaptive toy play modeled if the child's actions become repetitive (Hoban, 1988). Chapter 8 discusses the special recreation needs of children who are technology-assisted.

Participation of the child's caregivers should be encouraged in the child's overall care as well as within the stimulation program. Caregiver involvement benefits both the caregivers and the child in terms of fostering caregiver-child bonding and developmental growth. When caregiver involvement is limited, programs such as Foster Grandparents can be incorporated within a rehabilitation unit because their sole focus is on attending to the children's comfort and support rather than medical needs.

Interpersonal Relationships

In effect, nurses often serve as surrogate primary caregivers as many caregivers are not able to be bed or cribside on a regular or extended basis following admission to a rehabilitation unit (Bendell Estroff, in press). In general, attachment to a surrogate caregiver can be enhanced if a warm and consistent relationship is provided to the child (Dalton & Kirkhart, 1985). One way to provide such a relationship is to schedule the same nurses to care for identical children as much as possible (Miles & Mathes, 1991); unit staff even recommend that one nurse per shift be assigned the role of primary caretaker for each patient.

Unfortunately, nursing staff frequently become a "cue" for aversive stimuli (e.g., invasive medical procedures), resulting in an increase in problematic behaviors (Cataldo et al., 1979). The reaction of nursing staff to child aversive behaviors is often anger and frustration, with reduced time spent with the child or time limited to caring for medical needs (Dalton & Kirkhart, 1985). Staff can learn to depersonalize children's general problematic behaviors, which can interfere with individual care or that of other children on the unit (Dalton & Kirkhart, 1985). Providing staff with a conceptual frame-work in which to view such behavior may be helpful; for example, the problematic behaviors might be deemed as developmental tasks, efforts to obtain attention, or as resulting from sensory deprivation.

Support of Caregivers

Another strategy for developing attachment is to increase par-ticipation of caregivers in the care of the child through provision of preparatory information before the youngster enters the unit and then offering "caregiver education" classes once the child has been admitted. Recommendations regarding preparatory information and admission to an ICU are applicable for children on a rehabilitation unit and to their caregivers. For instance, preparatory information should be repeated and varied in focus, but should always include aspects of the caregiver-child relationship that may be changed during the admission (Miles & Mathes, 1991). Education of caregivers should emphasize both acquisition of information and skills. "Normal" developmental aspects or characteristics of the child should be discussed with the caregivers during visits and telephone contacts rather than only medical parameters (e.g., blood oxygen saturation levels). Discussion and training of the child's medical needs and care should be reserved for times other than when addressing develop-mental characteristics; these discussions should, however, focus on increasing caregiver knowledge of multiple aspects of their child. Caregivers should also be encouraged and assisted in learning the routine care of their child in terms of dressing and feeding; in general, attention should be given to well-baby care as well as to the special needs of the child. Various family issues, including preparatory information and stress of admissions, are explored in Chapter 10.

Play

Normalization of the environment through social interactions and provision of play materials has been proposed to prevent the traumatic effects of hospitalization (Blumgart & Korsch, 1964; Hott, 1970). Scheduled play activities should be incorporated into each child's daily routine, with both educational and creative toys provided as well as time with a caregiver or health care provider to stimulate play and socialization skills (see Chapter 8). In the study by Cataldo and colleagues (1979), an intervention involving planned play-related activities was evaluated following the observational assessment. Twelve children were observed during a series of conditions: "no toys," "toys available," and "person + toys." The activity intervention (especially the latter condition) resulted in increased interaction with toys or person, attention, and positive affect, plus decreased frequency of inappropriate behaviors (e.g., constant finger sucking, playing with EEG electrodes). However, the authors indicate that although the positive outcome of such planned activities is fairly apparent, the implementation and feasibility for specific hospital units is less clear.

Self-Help Skills

Another strategy that focuses on normalizing the environment of children who are technology-assisted is to teach or enhance self-care skills and/or adaptive behaviors. Depending on medical and maturational factors, such self-care skills as toileting and feeding could be taught to each child to increase their functional independence and socialization in preparation for discharge. Effective programs are available on toilet training and alleviation of enuresis in children with and without concomitant developmental delays (see Azrin & Foxx, 1971; Azrin, Sneed, & Foxx, 1974). Procedures to develop feeding skills are described in Chapter 5. Overall, the procedures used to teach these self-care skills and others (e.g., dressing, grooming) seem to have the following characteristics: reinforcement (social and tangible), prompting, chaining and shaping, time-out, and multiple but brief training sessions (Neisworth & Madle, 1982).

Behavioral Interventions

Influence of Environment

The literature suggests that environments that are dull, unvaried, and sparse in social interaction opportunities are likely to restrict repertoires of behavior (e.g., self-care skills, emotional-social reactions) (Neisworth & Madle, 1982). In addition, such environments tend to be unresponsive to adaptive behaviors and erratic in ignoring aberrant behaviors (Mace et al., 1992). As a result, extreme behaviors (e.g., disconnecting tubing from ventilators) may be shaped by a child to gain attention from adults (staff) in the environment (Mace et al., 1992). Another characteristic of sparse environments (or those that provide minimal opportunities for learning new skills) is inadequate reinforcement for task completion (e.g., dressing) or for engagement in social interactions (Mace et al., 1992).

Intervention Procedures

Numerous procedures are available that can successfully modify incidents of aberrant behaviors, especially self-stimulatory, self-injurious, and disruptive behaviors: time-out (removing child from source of attention contingent on occurrence of aberrant behavior), extinction (i.e., ignoring child following episode of aberrant behavior, which includes withholding social disapproval and reassurance comments), withholding access to tangible rewards or activities contingent on aberrant behavior, and overcorrection and positive practice. However, these procedures should be coupled with reinforcement techniques to develop and shape adaptive behaviors in the child, including increasing the rate of noncontingent attention and opportunities for social interactions, differentially reinforcing behaviors other than aberrant responses or behaviors incompatible with these behaviors (e.g., provide access to tangible rewards and activities contingent on occurrence of prosocial behaviors or approximation thereof), and teaching adaptive communicative responses for the child to obtain attention.

The following strategies (some of which were incorporated in the treatment of Monica, described below) can be employed to remediate aberrant behaviors on a rehabilitation unit, if such behaviors allow the child to escape or avoid aversive/demand situations: reducing task difficulty in combination with training those skills necessary to complete more difficult tasks, prompts or instructions to complete one part of a task at a time along with presentation of preferred activity, extinction (e.g., nonescape from task, guided compliance), and reinforcement for on-task behavior as well as for task completion. Finally, occurrence of self-stimulatory and self-injurious behaviors may be an attempt by the child to either amplify or reduce sensory input arising from sensory constraints imposed by the environment or a physical condition (Mace et al., 1992). Treatment strategies available to modify incidents of aberrant behavior consist of sensory extinction and environment enrichment (e.g., social interactions and activities) (Mace et al., 1992).

At present, there are no published studies of the implementation or the effectiveness of these procedures on the treatment of aberrant behaviors in children who are technology-assisted. However, the research indicates, in similar settings and with almost identical behaviors, the most effective treatment strategies (in terms of treatment gains and least reliance on aversive procedures) appear to be reinforcement techniques (especially differential reinforcement of incompatible behaviors), time-out, and overcorrection or extinction (Neisworth & Madle, 1982). Use of such punishment procedures as physical restraints and aversive aromas or tastes is not recommended because of ethics and uncertainty of the effect on children who are technology-assisted. On the other hand, these procedures should not be dismissed entirely, as the measures can lead to rapid abatement of serious aberrant behavior, as when, for example, the child's behavior is life-threatening and all other treatment procedures have been unsuccessful in decreasing or eliminating the behavior.

Mediating Variables

Several factors need to be considered before implementing the above procedures. For example, designation of a time-out area might not be possible for children connected to a ventilator who cannot be removed easily to another area. In addition, these children spend most of the day in their rooms, where they are bathed, dressed, fed, and put to bed; using the same area for all activities results in little if any discrimination for the child when they are in "time-out" versus "time-in." Another issue involves the ability of staff to ignore episodes of aberrant behaviors, such as self-decannulation or disconnection of the tubing. Nursing staff cannot ignore such behavior because of obvious medical reasons; thus, such behavior can be expected to garner consistent attention from all staff. However, staff can be instructed not to converse at all with the child and to give only the amount of time with the child necessary to ensure medical safety. Also to be considered is the number of training sessions and the total time required to produce meaningful treatment gains. Individuals designated to implement the treatment procedures, as well as means and scheduling for these individuals to be trained in the procedures, need to be determined.

Case Studies

The case of Sandy illustrates the use of behavioral techniques to treat severe self-stimulation, and that of Monica illustrates the use of social interactions and therapy activities to reduce incidents of abberant behavior.

Sandy

A 33-month-old former preemie diagnosed with chronic respiratory failure and developmental delays in the severe to profound range, Sandy engaged in a high rate of self-stimulatory behaviors, such as hand waving near her eyes, finger twirling, and tube biting (ventilator and gastrostomy tube). A protocol was devised to both increase manipulation of toys and decrease tube biting. The protocol focused on using a hands-down procedure after every episode of tube biting. That is, Sandy's hands were held at her sides or in front of her for 3-5 seconds, then she was guided in manipulating a toy for 10-15 seconds, as the actions with the toy were described to her. This protocol was implemented by staff during all therapies and routine care on the unit, as well as during daily sessions with a pediatric psychology intern. Partial success was achieved in substituting toy play for tube biting.

Monica

A 5-year-old child with multiple congenital anomalies and developmental delays in the moderate range who was ventilator-assisted, Monica emitted a variety of problematic behaviors, such as aggression toward staff (e.g. biting, scratching), and herself (e.g. head hitting) and disconnecting herself from the ventilator, along with limited prosocial behaviors. A comprehensive treatment plan was developed to both shape adaptive behaviors and reduce the incidence of aberrant behaviors. All staff were requested to implement the treatment plan, but consistency was difficult because of the sheer number of professionals involved in Monica's care. The plan included providing differential attention for adaptive/prosocial behaviors and interactions, fading of people and activities during transitional periods, structuring tasks and teaching sessions to heighten discrimination between time periods and activities, training in the use of a communication board to ease and enhance interactions, ignoring minor misbehaviors, and time-out for aggressive behaviors that was expanded from 1-minute to 5-minutes. The treatment plan was effective in significantly reducing the frequency and intensity of Monica's problematic behaviors and in fostering positive interactions between herself and the staff.

ROLE OF THE PSYCHOLOGIST WITH OTHER MEMBERS OF THE HEALTH CARE TEAM

The pediatric psychologist is well-positioned to make a significant contribution to children receiving technology assistance and their families, directly through personal contacts and indirectly through a consultative role with the health care staff.

The Psychologist and the Family

The psychologist's role will vary over time and across families, depending on the medical condition of the child and the needs and wants of individual families (Dalton & Kirkhart, 1985). Family needs in the acute stage of treatment, when life and death issues prevail, will differ from those in the transition to home stage. In the former, the psychologist can play a supportive role, helping the caregivers through the trauma of diagnosis, the decision to begin the ventilation, and the fears around their child's survival.

Later, in the intermediate and rehabilitative stages, when the child's medical condition is stable, other issues emerge that can be difficult for caregivers to manage, and if left unaddressed, can interfere with the child's long-term functioning. During this stage (which can last from days to years) caregivers might be coping with the loss of an idealized healthy infant, uncertainty around the child's future physical and psychological health, ambivalent feelings toward the child, and the challenge of developing a relationship with a child to whom they have limited access. At the same time, other family concerns continue. Extended family members must be managed, siblings need attention, jobs must be kept, a house maintained. If the hospital is outside the local community, visits involve extended absence from home and work, babysitting arrangements for other children, and additional financial strain. Any one of these issues can strain a family's emotional resources; in combination, they can be overwhelming.

Clinical reports and research data indicate that hospitalization of a child is stressful for both caregivers and the sick child (Knafl, Cavallari, & Dixon, 1988; King & Ziegler, 1981). Children who are technology-assisted and their caregivers are confronted with stressful events throughout the hospitalization, beginning in the ICU, moving to the rehabilitation unit, and continuing after discharge to either a long-term care facility or home. Aspects of the ICU stressful for the caregivers and the child include adjustment to strange surroundings and personnel, the sights and sounds of the units, invasive medical procedures done to the child, separation from family and friends, staff communication and behavior, and, perhaps most importantly, the child's emotional response and behavior plus alterations in the caregiver role (Miles & Mathes, 1991; Vernon, Foley, Sipowicz, & Schulman, 1965).

The psychologist can help the family identify these and other stresses, process their feelings, communicate among themselves, and strengthen support systems. The psychologist may also help care-givers find their place in their child's life in the hospital and facilitate the development of a meaningful caregiver-child relationship. Working directly with the child and family, the psychologist can interpret the child's cues, explain the youngster's needs in relation to developmental level, and facilitate the development of a reciprocal relationship. As the time nears for the child to leave the hospital, the psychologist can help the family process their fears and hopes around the transition. The psychologist can stay involved with the family as they take on the responsibility of caring for their child, managing home-care staff, and adjusting their existing household to accommodate the addition of a new family member, and medical equipment and nursing support. Later, the psychologist can help in promoting the child's mainstreaming into the classroom setting.

The Psychologist and Other Health Care Providers

The behavior of hospitalized children and their caregivers can appear confusing and destructive to the health care providers who have worked so hard to care for patient and family. Previously cooperative children (and their caregivers) can become resistant and angry. The psychologist can reframe this behavior to help hospital staff understand its roots and manage such occurrences more effectively (Dalton & Kirkhart, 1985; Hayes & Knox, 1984). Along with the social worker (see Chapter 10), the psychologist is positioned to be a liaison between the staff and family, seeking additional information, clarifying needs and concerns, interpreting feelings and behavior. Moreover, the psychologist can advocate for the caregivers in their attempts to define roles for themselves in the ongoing care of their child.

Role Conflicts

One stress source can be incongruence between health profes-sionals' view of the caregivers' role in hospital care and the caregivers' self-conception (Hayes & Knox, 1984). Open and honest communication between the caregivers and staff assists in develop-ing a trusting relationship, with concerns and questions addressed with little disruption to the family and to the unit (Bendell Estroff, in press; Hayes & Knox, 1984). Negotiation of mutually acceptable roles in the care of the child can then occur, which will presumably ease stress in the caregivers and the staff (Hayes & Knox, 1984). Along these lines, a liaison, other than nursing or medical staff, should be available to assist in negotiations and to serve as a link between the family and various hospital systems.

Ongoing communication can also be a mechanism for sharing general information beyond addressing concerns. For example, the nursing staff can provide caregivers valuable information about specific characteristics of the child (e.g., sensitivity to touch, favored sleeping position) as well as developmental aspects (e.g., when began to track, youngster's weight). In turn, such sharing of information will expand the caregivers' role in child care and, as a result, alleviate some of the stress experienced by nursing staff (Bendell Estroff, in press).

Common strategies to reduce stress felt by various hospital staff consist of peer support through education and discussion (Bendell Estroff, in press). Providing a forum for staff to discuss their views and concerns about individual children can help in decreasing burnout rate and in improving job satisfaction (Hayes & Knox, 1984). For example, medical support groups led by a pediatric psychologist, psychiatrist, or social worker; in-services for hospital staff with periodic "booster" sessions; and/or workshops with ongoing discussion groups led by staff themselves are several forums for educational and emotional support.

CONCLUSIONS

Children with long-term tracheostomies and their families face a complex array of medical, developmental, and behavioral challenges. Awareness of these potential problems and their relationship to typical development can prepare caregivers and health care personnel to respond to these challenges more effectively. This chapter presented issues related to etiology, assessment, and intervention for developmental and behavior problems in children who have undergone long-term hospitalization. Enhancing cognitive, social, and emotional development should be an essential goal in treatment planning for children with tracheostomies. Such comprehensive programming entails careful coordination between members of the health care team.

REFERENCES

Ainsworth, M., Bell, S., & Stayton, D. (1974). Infant-mother attachment and social development: Socialization as a product of reciprocal responsiveness to signals. In M.J.M. Richards (Ed.), *The integration of a child into a social world* (pp. 99-136). London: Cambridge University Press.

Ainsworth, M., & Bowlby, J. (1991). An ethnological approach to personality development. *American Psychologist, 46(4),* 333-341.

Azrin, N.H., & Foxx, R.M. (1971). A rapid method of toilet training the institutionalized retarded. *Journal of Applied Behavior Analysis, 4,* 89-99.

Azrin, N.H., Sneed, T.J., & Foxx, R.M. (1974). Dry bed training: Rapid elimination of childhood enuresis. *Behavior Research and Therapy, 12,* 147-156.

Ball, R.S., Merrifield, P., & Stott, L.H. (1978). *Extended Merrill-Palmer Scale.* Chicago: Stoelting.

Bayley, N. (1969). *Bayley Scales of Infant Development: Birth to two years.* New York: Psychological Corporation.

Bell, S. M., & Ainsworth, M.D.S. (1972). Infant crying and maternal responsiveness. *Child Development, 43,* 1171-1190.

Bendell Estroff, D. (in press). The pediatric psychologist and the N.I.C.U. In R.A. Olson & L.L. Mullins (Eds.), *Pediatric psychology handbook.* Baltimore: Johns Hopkins.

Blumgart, E., & Korsch, B.M. (1964). Pediatric recreation: An approach to meeting the emotional needs of hospitalized children. *Pediatrics, 34,* 133-136.

Bowlby, J. (1960). Separation anxiety. *International Journal of Psychoanalysis, 41,* 89-113.

Bowlby, J. (1961). Separation anxiety: A critical review of the literature. *Journal of Child Psychology and Psychiatry, 1,* 251- 269.

Bronfenbrenner, U. (1979). *The ecology of human development: Experiments by nature and design.* Cambridge, Harvard University Press.

Carr, E.G. (1977). The motivation of self-injurious behavior: A review of some hypotheses. *Psychological Bulletin, 84,* 800-816.

Cataldo, M.F., Bessman, C.A., Parker, L.H., Pearson, J.E., & Rogers, M.C. (1979). Behavioral assessment for pediatric intensive care units. *Journal of Applied Behavior Analysis, 12,* 83-97.

Cataldo, M.F., Jacobs, H.E., & Rogers, M.C. (1982). Behavioral/environmental considerations in pediatric inpatient care. In D.C. Russo & J.W. Varni (Eds.), *Behavioral pediatrics. Research and practice* (pp. 271-298). New York: Plenum Press.

Dalton, R., & Kirkhart, K. (1985, winter). An evolution of emotional problems faced by ventilator-assisted children. *The Pediatric Forum,* 73-81.

Erickson, E. (1963). *Childhood and society.* New York: Norton.

Foster, S.L., & Cone, J.D. (1980). Current issues in direct observation. *Behavioral Assessment, 2,* 313-338.

Gorski, P.A. (1983). Premature infant behavioral and physiological response to care giving interventions in the intensive care nursery. In J. Call, E. Galenson, & R. Tyson (Eds.), *Frontiers of infant psychiatry* (pp. 256-263). New York: Basic Books.

Hayes, V.E., & Knox, J.E. (1984). The experience of stress in parents of children hospitalized with long-term disabilities. *Journal of Advanced Nursing, 9,* 333-341.

Haynes, S.N., & Jensen, B.J. (1979). The interview as a behavioral assessment instrument. *Behavioral Assessment, 1,* 97-106.

Haynes, S.N., & Wilson, C.C. (1979). *Behavioral assessment: Recent advances in methods, concepts, and applications.* San Francisco: Jossey-Bass.

Hoban, S. (1988). Attention and memory. In N.R. Bartel, V.C. Peckham, & J. Radcliffe (Eds.), *Educational handbook for parents of preschool children with brain tumors.* Unpublished manuscript.

Hott, J. (1970). Rx: Play PRN in pediatric nursing. *Nursing, 9,* 288-309.

Ilg, F.L., & Ames, L.B. (1965). *School readiness: Behavior tests used at the Gesell Institute.* New York: Harper & Row.

Jones, R.R., Reid, J.B., & Patterson, G.R. (1975). Naturalistic observation in clinical assessment. In P. McReynolds (Ed.), *Advances in psychological assessment* Vol. 3 (pp. 42-95). San Francisco: Jossey-Bass.

Kanfer, F.H., & Saslow, G. (1969). Behavioral diagnosis. In C. M. Franks (Ed.), *Behavior therapy: Appraisal and status* (pp. 417-444). New York: McGraw-Hill.

King, J., & Ziegler, S. (1981). The effects of hospitalization on children's behavior: A review of the literature. *Children's Health Care, 10,* 20-28.

Knafl, K.A., Cavallari, K.A., & Dixon, D.M. (1988). *Pediatric hospitalization: Family and nurse perspectives.* Glenview, IL: Scott, Foresman, & Co.

Lerner, R. (1987). The concept of plasticity in development. In J.J. Gallagher & C.T. Ramey (Eds.), *The malleability of children* (pp. 3-14). Baltimore: Paul H. Brookes.

Linehan, M.M. (1977). Issues in behavioral interviewing. In J.D. Cone & R.P. Hawkins (Eds.), *Behavioral assessment: New directions in clinical psychology* (pp. 30-51). New York: Brunner/Mazel.

Lowe, M. (1975). Trends in the development of representational play in infants from one to three years—An observational study. *Journal of Child Psychology and Psychiatry, 16,* 33-47.

Lowe, M., & Costello, A.J. (1976). *Manual of the Symbolic Play Test.* Windsor, Berks, England: NFER.

Mace, F.C., Lalli, J.S., & Shea, M.C. (1992). Functional analysis and treatment of self-injury. In J. Luiselli, J. Matson, & N. Singh (Eds.), *Assessment, analysis, and treatment of self-injury* (pp. 122-152). New York: Springer-Verlag.

Mash, E.J., & Terdal, L.G. (1981). Behavioral assessment of childhood disturbance. In E.J. Mash & L.G. Terdal (Eds.), *Behavioral assessment of childhood disorders* (pp. 3-76). New York: Guilford Press.

Miles, M.S., & Mathes, M. (1991). Preparation of parents for the ICU experience: What are we missing? *Children's Health Care, 20,* 132-137.

Neisworth, J.T., & Madle, R.A. (1982). Retardation. In A.S. Bellack, M. Hersen, & A.E. Kazdin (Eds.), *International handbook of behavior modification and therapy* (pp. 853-889). New York: Plenum Press.

Nelson, R.O., & Hayes, S.C. (1979). Some current dimensions of behavioral assessment. *Behavioral Assessment, 1,* 1-16.

Ollendick, T.H., & Hersen, M. (1984). An overview of child behavioral assessment. In T.H. Ollendick & M. Hersen (Eds.), *Child behavioral assessment. Principles and procedures* (pp. 3-19). New York: Pergamon Press.

Piaget, J. (1967). *Play, dreams, and imitation in childhood* (C. Gattegno & F.M. Hodgson, Trans.). New York: Norton. (Original work published 1947).

Sameroff, A. (1981). Longitudinal studies of preterm infants. In S.L. Friedman & M. Sigman (Eds.), *Preterm birth and psychological development.* New York: Academic Press.

Sameroff, A., & Chandler, M. (1975). Reproductive risk and the continuum of caretaking casualty. In F.D. Horowitz (Ed.) *Review of child development research, Vol. 4.* Chicago: University of Chicago Press.

Sattler, J.M. (1988). *Assessment of children (3rd ed.).* San Diego, CA: Jerome M. Sattler, Publisher.

Seligman, M.E.P. (1991). *Helplessness: On development, depression, and death.* San Francisco: W.H. Freeman & Co.

Spitz, R. (1945). Anaclitic depression. *Psychoanalytic study of the child, 2,* 313-392.

Stern, D. (1974). The goal and structure of mother-infant play. *Journal of the American Academy of Child Psychiatry, 13,* 408-421.

Thoman, E. (1987). Self-regulation of stimulation by prematures with a breathing blue bear. In J.J. Gallagher & C.T. Ramey (Eds.), *The malleability of children.* Baltimore: Paul H. Brookes.

Thorndike, R.L., Hagen, E.P., & Sattler, J.M. (1986). *Guide for administering and scoring the Stanford-Binet Intelligence Scale:* 4th Edition. Chicago: Riverside Publishing.

Tizard, B., & Hodges, J. (1978). The effect of early institutional rearing on the development of eight year old children. *Journal of Child Psychology and Psychiatry, 19,* 99-118.

Tizard, B., & Rees, J. (1975). The effect of early institutional rearing on the behavioral problems and affectional relationships of four year old children. *Journal of Child Psychology and Psychiatry, 16,* 61-73.

Vernon, D.T., Foley, J.M., Sipowicz, R.R., & Schulman, J.L. (1965). *The psychological responses of children to hospitalization and illness: A review of the literature.* Springfield, IL: Charles Thomas Publishers.

Wechsler, D. (1989). *Manual for the Wechsler preschool and primary scale of intelligence—revised.* New York: Psychological Corp.

Yarrow, L., Rubenstein, J., & Pedersen, F. (1975). *Infant and environment: Early cognitive and motivational development.* Washington, DC: Hemisphere.

8

Recreation

Mary Ann Caromano Roberto

INTRODUCTION

Intervention for a child with a **tracheostomy** does not stop at the door of the therapy room. Instead, developmentally appropriate recreation activities are incorporated into both the child's daily routines and play. This chapter discusses recreation activities for young children with **long-term tracheostomies.** The following topics are addressed:

• The role of play in development
• Hospital recreation groups
• Other hospital recreation programs
• Community-based recreation programs and resources
• Using recreation activities to help with care location transitions
• The role of therapeutic recreation

THE ROLE OF RECREATION IN DEVELOPMENT

Recreation is important because of its role in children's development. For example, when a child builds a tower of blocks the youngster facilitates development of speech, language, motor skills, cognition, and socialization. To illustrate, by saying "block" to ask for a block from an adult sitting nearby, the child practices speech and language. As the child puts one block on another, the youngster is developing eye-hand coordination and fine motor skills. When knocking down the block tower, the child is learning about cause-and-effect relationships. By helping put the blocks away when play is over, the child is acquiring social rules.

Recreation activities for children with long-term tracheostomies are designed to provide children opportunities for play, learning, self-expression, family involvement, and peer interactions. Recreation is also intended to enable the child and caregivers to adjust to and cope with anxieties, fears, and uncertainties related to the child's disability and limited mobility (Greenspan & Greenspan, 1985).

HOSPITAL RECREATION GROUPS

Recreation can be with an individual child or in a group, at bedside or in a recreation area. This section describes the purposes and procedures of hospital recreation groups. The hospital group activities described might easily be adapted to one-on-one play between a child and an adult, either in a hospital setting or in the community.

Goals

The general purpose of a hospital recreation group is to provide a structured daily program of activities facilitating the development of communication and functional skills across areas of play, socialization, self-care, motor development, and educational readiness. The following are the therapeutic objectives of recreation groups:

1. Establish and maintain a consistent routine for implementation of daily programmatic functions;
2. Facilitate the child's awareness of the people and objects in the environment;
3. Facilitate development in the areas of sensory stimulation (auditory, visual, tactile, olfactory, taste), and development in the areas of fine and gross motor skills, communication, cognition, and socialization; and
4. Expose the child to new experiences.

Populations

Recreation groups are beneficial to all children, especially those with known developmental disabilities as well as those at-risk for developmental delays secondary to chronic illness, prolonged hospitalization, or family difficulties in adapting to the stress of a child with a disability. Both Lisa and Frank (see Chapter 1 for introductory case history) are excellent candidates for recreation groups.

Referrals

Children are referred to recreation groups by therapeutic recreation specialists, physicians, nurses, social workers, or therapists. To promote the best care for the child, the referral includes information on the child's level of functioning in social and emotional development, cognition, communication, gross motor and fine motor skills, and self-help skills. The referral should also note any special limitations or restrictions a child may have. Adapted devices or equipment may also be requested. Appendix 8-A contains a sample referral form.

Assessment

In addition to the information in the referral, an assessment should be undertaken to determine the likely degree of caregiver involvement in the child's program, the child's level of responsiveness to various toys and activities, and the youngster's general level of development in the following areas: communication, cognition, behavior, emotional development, motor skills, leisure activities, and socialization. The assessment is based on interviews with the child and guardians, direct interaction with the child, and observation of the child's play. Possible activities that might be used in the assessment of play include reading to the child, sharing a special book or toy, or simply talking to the child about herself, family, or everyday activities.

Location

Playrooms in hospitals must be specially designed for the child with a tracheostomy, especially if the child is also oxygen or **ventilator-assisted.** Special oxygen, air, suction, and electrical outlets need to be built into wall structures or into custom-designed play tables constructed to accommodate a child's height. Open floor areas need to be sufficiently large to accommodate ventilators, monitors, and various emergency equipment. Additionally, for the playroom to appeal to the child, necessary medical equipment should be surrounded by brilliant colors and interesting forms and textures. Toy shelves (out of the reach of the children) should contain baskets of rattles, textured objects, blocks, mirrors, shape sorters, cause-effect toys, adaptive switch and plate toys, art materials, and educational games. Larger play materials, including varying sized balls, tunnels, rocking horses and boats, riding toys, and tricycles, can be placed in corners of the room. Petite tables, chairs, therapeutic adaptive tables, corner seats, sidelyers, prone standers, and standing boxes should be available at all times.

Organization

Recreation groups should be divided into infant, toddler, and preschool groups. Groups are held 1 to 3 times daily for 1 to 2 hours. Generally, children functioning developmentally between 0 to 7 months are placed in the infant group, children functioning developmentally from between 8 to 18 months and from 19 to 30 months are placed in toddler groups, and children functioning between 30 to 60 months are placed in the preschool groups. Approximately 5 to 8 children should be in each program.

Recreation groups may contain three segments: Circle Time, Table Time, and Active Play. Each segment has specific therapeutic interventions and activities for the children in the group. Additionally, each child has individual rehabilitative goals and objectives. Although the goals of each segment are generally the same among the groups, the activities obviously vary as a function of the developmental level of the children in the group.

Prior to Group

Before beginning a group session, large play mats are arranged in the center of the playroom floor. The transfer of the children from their rooms is facilitated by respiratory therapy and nursing staffs to assure proper equipment functioning and the safety of the environment.

Circle Time

Circle Time focuses on communication development, cognitive stimulation, and socialization. In an interdisciplinary group, the discipline likely to have primary responsibility for Circle Time is speech-language pathology. Circle Time typically begins with a "Hello" song. After identifying and welcoming each child, interactive songs are performed by the therapists and children in the group. The therapists provide hand-over-hand assistance to children as needed, maximizing each child's level of participation. At the close of Circle Time, a song called "Circle Time Is Over" may be performed.

Table Time

Table Time provides an opportunity for children to handle various textures, arts and craft materials, and manipulative playthings. In addition to promoting fine motor skills, Table Time provides opportunities for interaction and communication. In an interdisciplinary group, the discipline likely to have primary responsibility for Table Time is occupational therapy. If preceded by Circle Time, this segment begins with the infant and toddler groups being encouraged to independently or with assistance crawl or ambulate to the table. Table Time ends with the children assisting in the clean-up process and washing their own hands and their table space.

Active Play

Active Play provides experience in gross motor skills. These experiences facilitate movement, vestibular coordination, and overall physical and respiratory endurance. In an interdisciplinary group, the discipline most likely to have primary responsibility for Active Play is physical therapy. Active Play begins with a warm up song to encourage stretching and body movement. During Active Play the children engage in such activities as rolling large therapeutic balls, jumping on an air mattress, riding toys, swimming in a pool of balls, and dancing. The session concludes with a snack of a popsicle or cookie, which encourages the handling of food and stimulation of the taste sense. Lastly, the children sing a "goodbye" song.

Transitional Times

After each segment, a transitional period is allotted for clean-up, walking, crawling, or transferring to the area for the next segment and for any nursing needs that may need to be addressed (for example, suctioning). Transitional periods last approximately 5 to 10 minutes. These periods must be brief to maintain a child's short attention span. In most infant groups, a transitional period is much shorter or nonexistent because the majority of activities are on a centrally located floor mat.

OTHER HOSPITAL RECREATION PROGRAMS

Other hospital recreation programs popular with children with tracheostomies include Story hour, Pet Therapy, Cooking with Kids, and the ABC's of Colors and Shapes, plus field trips. To facilitate peer awareness and interaction, these programs should include opportunities for children with tracheostomies to interact both with each other and with other children.

Program Ideas

Story Hour

Story hour provides toddlers and preschoolers 1-hour sessions focusing on interactive play and self-expression. Story hour should be held in a quiet room with minimal stimuli. Ideal group size is 4 to 6 children. Selected stories should be brief and geared toward the cognitive level of the group. Typically, a story is told using felt board activities, puppets, finger plays, or other objects.

Pet Therapy

Pet Therapy appeals to children of all ages. Pet Therapy addresses goals in sensory stimulation and in psychosocial and emotional development. In planning a Pet Therapy program, special consideration needs to be given to health codes, allergies, and children's behavior and fears. Before the pets arrive, the location where the pets will be placed needs to be identified. Supervised groups of 2 to 4 children are rotated to see and touch the animals. To avoid possible difficulties, the program should utilize Certified Pet Therapy animals to assure the good health, training, and temperament of the animal.

Cooking With Kids

Cooking with Kids appeals to preschoolers and school-aged children. Cooking with Kids provides opportunity for socialization, development of fine motor and communication skills, and the promotion of activities of daily living. Children referred to this program must be able to tolerate a 1-hour session, demonstrate self-control, follow one-step directions, and be able to communicate their basic needs. An adult to child ratio of 1:3 and a maximum group size of 6 children enables close supervision and assistance for each child. A cooking group skills assessment form such as that in Appendix 8-B can be used to monitor ongoing cooking skills acquisition.

ABCs of Colors and Shapes

The ABCs of Colors and Shapes program is appropriate for toddlers and preschool-age children. For this activity, children are provided materials and situations to facilitate identification of colors, shapes, perceptual concepts, sharing, taking turns during interactions, following simple task directives, and problem solving. Group size may vary depending on each child's independence level. The maximum group size is 8 children. The physical environment should allow each child to clearly see the therapist and to have adequate table workspace. Activity materials should be prepared before the session begins and need to be easily accessible to maintain a steady flow of stimulation for the children.

Field Trips

Field Trips offer valuable experiences for children of all ages. If the child is residing in a hospital, Field Trips provide good opportunities for families to prepare for family life beyond the secure care of around-the-clock physicians and nurses.

Field Trips are typically developed in collaboration with hospital staff and the family. At first, even brief strolls around the building provide an abundance of sensory experience to a young child. If the child has never or seldom been in an outdoor environment, the sights and sounds of cars, the touch of grass, rocks, and trees, and even varying temperatures may be intimidating and sometimes frightening. Caregivers are strongly encouraged to join their child during these brief initial outings both because the walks provide caregivers and child opportunities to share in a child's first new experiences and because Field Trips provide excellent opportunities for the family to become involved in the care and management of their child. Brief strolls around the building eventually lead to half-day and then full-day trips into the community. These longer Field Trips may include visits to such childhood attractions as playgrounds, parks, zoos, children's museums, community theaters, and even amusement parks.

COMMUNITY-BASED RECREATION PROGRAMS

Although far from common, there are some excellent community-based medically fragile programs and specially designed summer camp programs for children with medical disabilities. Medically fragile programs are structured similarly to early intervention programs. These programs provide services to children with tracheostomies, including those requiring oxygen and ventilatory support.

At least two organizations offer summer camps for children receiving ventilator assistance. These are the Miami Children's

Hospital Ventilator-Assisted Children's Center (VACC) Camp and SKIP (Sick Kids Need Involved People) Camp. The book Appendix lists the addresses of both camps. Both organizations offer a 1-week summer camp for children receiving ventilator assistance and their families. These camps provide opportunity for children to come together with others like themselves and to participate in a variety of childhood activities, including day trips, movies, campfires, story-telling, arts and crafts, and fishing trips. The camps are staffed by physicians, nurses, respiratory therapists, educators, and nutritionists. In addition to providing excellent experiences to the children, the camps give caregivers the opportunity to share similar experiences, and exchange support, suggestions, resources, and encouragements.

Lastly, many community recreational facilities, parks, YMCAs, and children's programs are accessible and available to children with disabilities, including those with tracheostomies and those receiving ventilator assistance. Local libraries and public schools can often identify other resources available in the community. If no suitable program exists, therapists may wish to consider developing one. An example of a successful annual event for young children with disabilities is the "Sesame Place Challenge for Variety Club," held annually in Langhorne, PA. The event promotes a family-centered day of fun-filled activity for children with disabilities and their siblings. Through healthy challenge and competition, children are provided the opportunity to "take the Sesame Place challenge" and experience fun, "normal" childhood activity in an environment safely designed and supported by volunteers of therapeutic professions under the direction of Sesame Place park employees. This program was developed through the efforts of the Philadelphia Variety Club, the Sesame Place Entertainment Facility, and a committee of representatives from children's hospitals, centers, and homes in the Philadelphia and surrounding area. The committee consists primarily of therapeutic recreation specialists.

TRANSITIONS

Recreation activities can play an important role in helping the child and caregivers with transitions from the acute care setting to the rehabilitation hospital, and, later, from the rehabilitation hospital to the community.

Transition From an Acute Care Unit

The transition from the acute care unit to a rehabilitation hospital is often difficult for the child and family—especially if the child has undergone long-term hospitalization. Although the hospital staff views such a change as recovery from illness, a child with a tracheostomy and the youngster's family might find this change a disruption of a once tolerable and even comfortable routine.

Before the child's transfer from the acute care setting, the recreation activities available in the new setting should be discussed with the child (when appropriate) and the youngster's caregivers. Many children and their families become reassured in hearing about the rehabilitation hospital's special playrooms, recreation areas, toys, games, and activities. A book of photographs may enable young children to look forward to an easier adjustment. Additional transition aids may include such objects as a soothing blanket for an infant or a special toy or book for an older child (Poster, 1985; Nesbitt, 1985). Caregivers should also be encouraged to visit the "new environment" prior to the transfer. Lastly, it is also important to establish behavioral limits for the child and daily routines for physical care, naps, and playtime. This should be established early in the transition phase with the child's caregivers.

Once the child is in the new setting, an important goal is to give the child a sense of comfort, trust, and control in the new environment. Interacting with the child at bedside may help give the child this sense of control. Early interactions might include brief verbal encounters, reading stories, sharing of a special toy, or decorating the bedside area. Hospital staff should not attempt to "rush" the new relationship with the child. This includes not touching or handling the child unless the child invites an adult to do so.

Transition to the Community

Discharge to home from the hospital may represent yet another transition and adjustment for child and family (Lawrence, 1984). This is because most young children with tracheostomies have been hospitalized all or most of their lives and only know a world surrounded by doctors, nurses, and medical machinery. Further, as in Frank's case, many caregivers, although excited that their child will be at home, may also be frightened and unsure of their ability to handle and care for their child's special needs (see Chapter 10). These caregivers require additional support, encouragement, and guidance in order to confidently and successfully fulfill their responsibilities. A percentage of young children with tracheostomies will be placed under the care of foster caregivers. These children need to be given ample time to "get-to-know" their new guardians.

As the discharge approaches, the guardians' home should be assessed for safety of the furniture and materials within the play space and for possible outdoor play opportunities. If there is no play area, a member of the hospital team should discuss how to convert existing spaces in the home and yard into play spaces. This assessment of the home is formulated into a suggestion sheet or plan for the family.

After the assessment is completed, a member of the hospital team needs to provide family counseling about play activities that may facilitate the child's growth and development. This counseling might include helping guardians select toys, find community resources, financial aid, or toy patterns to make, talking with the family about play safety issues and discussing how to avoid overstimulating the child during play. As part of this discussion, families might be offered selected articles, brochures, and books. Possible community-based recreation services for the family should also be identified.

At the time of discharge, a packet should be prepared for the community-based day care center or other educational or recreational program the child may be entering. Appendix 8-C lists the information that should be included in such a packet, including the hospital recreation goals and course of intervention. The packet should also describe the child's affect, interactive skills, personality, emotional response to various environmental stimuli, and the child's response to preferred and nonpreferred recreational activities and experiences. Additionally, the packet should contain specific suggestions for community interventions.

Lastly, just before discharge the hospital team often plan a "send-off" party for the child and family. The party is offered by all disciplines involved with the child throughout the hospitalization. This party often reassures the family of the love and support that the hospital staff have committed to sharing with them.

THE ROLE OF THERAPEUTIC RECREATION

In many settings the discipline most directly responsible for developing recreation activities is therapeutic recreation. Therapeutic recreation activities are designed to restore, remediate, or rehabilitate functioning and independence as well as reduce or eliminate the effects of illness or disability. Therapeutic recreation specialists make adaptations to recreational activities, toys, and the environment to maximize the child's level of participation in everyday leisure experiences. Therapeutic recreation specialists work closely with occupational therapy, psychiatry, physical therapy, nursing, social work, psychology, and speech-language pathology. Additionally, therapeutic recreation specialists have close contact with the child's caregivers to encourage caregiver and sibling involvement in the child's programs both before and after hospital discharge.

Goals

The following are overall therapeutic recreation goals:

1. Identify individualized needs of children and remediate specific areas of difficulty;
2. Provide play and recreational opportunities promoting physical, social, emotional, and language development;
3. Provide leisure awareness, education, and counselling to the child and caregivers;
4. Identify and provide the child and caregivers with community resources;
5. Assist caregivers in developing skills in managing the child's developmental, communicative, and daily needs; and
6. Offer an integrated, holistic, and family-centered program of developmental intervention.

Therapeutic Recreation Activities

Therapeutic recreation activities are beneficial in promoting sensory stimulation and development of motor skills, communication, cognition, and socialization. Table 8-1 lists activities used to meet these therapeutic objectives.

As the information in Table 8-1 suggests, auditory stimulation is facilitated through the introduction of manipulative toys capable of producing sounds. Examples of such toys are rattles, activity centers, and musical instruments. Visual stimulation is encouraged by creating an environment with a variety of colors. The facilitation of tactile stimulation is developed through activities involving objects with a variety of different textures. Useful substances for this include water, Playdoh, sandpaper, and cotton. Useful food substances include flour, raw or cooked noodles, peanut butter, pudding, and oatmeal.

Stimulation of the olfactory sense is facilitated through activities involving different spices, extracts, sweet and sour substances, and everyday household items such as nontoxic soaps, nonaerosol air fresheners, and perfumes. The development of a taste response is often delayed in young children who are tracheostomized because they are likely to have been fed via nasogastric tubes, gastrostomy

TABLE 8-1. Areas of development facilitated through therapeutic recreation activities.

AREA OF THERAPY	ACTIVITY
Auditory stimulation	Shaking rattle Operating activity center Playing musical instrument
Visual stimulation	Color variation in environment Novel visual textures
Tactile stimulation	Playing with water, Playdoh, sandpaper, and cotton, as well as with food substances such as flour, raw or cooked noodles, peanut butter, pudding, and oatmeal
Olfactory stimulation	Smelling spices, extracts, sweet and sour substances, and other everyday household items such as non-toxic soaps, air fresheners, and perfumes
Taste stimulation	Tasting various foods
Motor development	Riding a tricycle Art projects Climbing stairs Jumping on a trampoline Crawling through a tunnel Rolling across a mat
Language, cognitive, and social development	All activities Sharing "reading" of books Telling and listening to stories with finger puppets Singing interactive songs Interactive games

tubes, or by other methods not involving eating by mouth. The therapeutic recreation specialist facilitates taste development by developing play with and taste of food.

Motoric deficits are addressed by the therapeutic recreation specialist through activities promoting fine and gross motor development. Examples of such activities include riding tricycles, climbing stairs, crawling or walking through an obstacle course, jumping on a trampoline, crawling through a tunnel, and rolling across a mat.

Development of communication, cognition, and socialization are incorporated into all therapeutic recreation activities. Specific play activities to promote development in these areas include telling stories with finger puppets, participating in interactive songs, and listening to and telling stories. Socialization is facilitated particularly well at meal time, rest periods, and during the child's many daily care routines.

Sequence of Activities

Therapeutic recreation typically organizes the above activities into active-passive-active-passive sequences. Alternating the activities helps to keep the child interested and avoids overstimulation. The following is an example of an alternating sequence of active-passive activities:

Active: The child rides a tricycle
Passive: The child sits at a table for an art project promoting fine motor development
Active: The child negotiates an obstacle course of climbing stairs, jumping on a trampoline, crawling through a tunnel, and rolling across a mat
Passive: The child eats a snack

Educational Themes

In many instances, recreation therapy builds lessons around themes. Possible themes include holidays, seasons of the year, and special events, as well as activities built around various colors, shapes, and objects. In addition to providing a means to organize lessons, themes are a means to provide a colorful and structured environment for the children, staff, families, and visitors.

An example of the development of a theme might be "October is Fall." One week, such a program might focus strictly on apples, including the shape of apples (round), the color of apples (red or green), as well as apple projects, one possibly being to color a picture of an apple. Circle Time might include songs about apples while passing apples around the circle and placing pictures of apples on a felt board. Table Time might include gluing apple-shaped felt and sandpaper cut-outs onto a prefabricated tree, red or green fingerpainting, or even mixing applesauce. Lastly, Active Play might include "swimming" in a pool of red or green balls, carrying or pushing a cart of apples across the room, or being rolled on a large red or green therapeutic ball.

CONCLUSIONS

Recreation activities bring developmental interventions "out of the therapy room" and into the child's play and daily routines. Within hospital settings, recreation groups and programs can be important means to encourage play and socialization to facilitate overall growth and development. In the community, organized recreational opportunities are found in day care centers and camps specially designed for children with disabilities. Recreation activities are also important in helping children and their caregivers during difficult transition periods, such as when the child is moving from an acute care setting to a rehabilitation hospital or from a rehabilitation hospital to the community. In many settings, therapeutic recreation is the discipline most directly responsible for the recreation needs of children with tracheostomies.

REFERENCES

Greenspan, S., & Greenspan, N.T. (1985). *First feelings: Milestones in the emotional development of your baby and child.* New York: Viking Penguin.

Lawrence, P. (1984). Home care for ventilator dependent children: providing a chance to live a normal life. *Dimensions of critical care nursing, 3,* 42-52.

Nesbitt, T. (1985). Psychosocial needs of infants and toddlers: Implications for care. In C. Fore & E. Poster (Eds.), *Meeting psychosocial needs of children and families in health care* (pp. 38-42). Washington, DC: Association for the Care of Children's Health.

Poster, E.C. (1985). Stress immunization techniques to promote behavioral and cognitive control in hospitalized children. In C. Fore & E. Poster (Eds.), *Meeting psychosocial needs of children and families in health care* (pp. 67-72). Washington, DC: Association for the Care of Children's Health.

APPENDIX 8-A

Referral for Hospital Recreation Group

Request for Specific Services

Patient: _____

Person/Dept. Making Request: _____

DOB/Age: _____

Reason for Request: _____

Diagnosis: _____

Are you or someone from your department able to participate in a program if needed? _____

Developmental Level of Functioning

Please list specific level and additional descriptive information as needed:

Social/Emotional:

Cognitive:

Language:

Gross Motor:

Fine Motor:

Self-Help:

Please list any adaptive equipment that the child currently uses for any activities throughout the day. _____

_____

Please list any pertinent medical information on special care or special equipment. (i.e., central line, tracheostomy, open wound, and so on.)

_____

Please note: This request form should be utilized by physicians, clinical therapies, and nursing staff.

APPENDIX 8-B

Cooking Group Skills Assessment

I. COMMUNICATION (Wants and Needs)

A. Verbal

_____

_____

B. Sign

_____

_____

C. Picture

_____

_____

II. SELF-HELP	*Child Can Do*	*Child Can't Do*
A. Washes hands & or face	_____	_____
B. Stirs with spoon	_____	_____
C. Cleans up after self	_____	_____
D. Washes hands in appropriate sequence with minimal assistance	_____	_____
E. Drinks from a glass using one hand	_____	_____
F. Pours from a small container into a glass w/assistance	_____	_____
G. Eats at the table requiring little adult attention	_____	_____
H. Begins using a fork to pierce food rather than scoop	_____	_____

	Child Can Do	Child Can't Do
I. Responsible for own belongings	_____	_____
J. Feeds self independently when food cut into bite size	_____	_____
K. Manipulates fork/spoon	_____	_____
L. Controls pouring	_____	_____
M. Cleans up spills	_____	_____
N. Spreads with knife	_____	_____
O. Can help others	_____	_____
P. Washes dishes	_____	_____
Q. Cuts with knife	_____	_____
R. Uses fork to cut food	_____	_____
S. Prepares simple food with minimal assistance	_____	_____

II. *AWARENESS OF ENVIRONMENT*

	Child Can Do	Child Can't Do
A. *Self-Protection Reflex*	_____	_____
B. *Sense of Danger*	_____	_____
1. Awareness of hot	_____	_____
2. Awareness of cold	_____	_____
3. Avoids common dangers (i.e., broken glass)	_____	_____
C. *Awareness of Physical Boundaries* (People, furniture, steps, walls, doors, windows, etc.)	_____	_____

Therapist Signature / Date

APPENDIX 8-C

Sample Discharge Checklist

Recreation Goals While in Hospital:

Child Affective Characteristics:

Interactive Skills:

Response to Environmental Stimuli:

Preferred Recreation Play Activities:

Nonpreferred Recreation Play Activities:

Suggestions for Intervention:

SECTION IV

CARE IN THE HOME

The Care of
Children c̄ Long-Term
Tracheostomies
Edited by: Ken M Bleile

Pub: Singular, Sandiego
1993

9

Legal Rights to Education Services

Deborah Kitley and Jennifer Buzby-Hadden

INTRODUCTION

This chapter describes the legal basis for providing educational services to children with tracheostomies. It is estimated that at the end of 1990 more than 600,000 children with special needs, birth through 5 years of age, were receiving intervention services in the United States (U.S. Department of Education, 1991). It is important for all health care providers to understand the legal rights for educational services of the children they serve. Although laws differ by state and care setting, there is a core of federal law pertaining to all children with developmental disabilities who receive services in the United States. This chapter describes those laws. The following topics are addressed:

• The legal rights of children 0-3 years to educational services
• The early intervention process for children from birth through 3 years of age
• The legal rights of children 3-21 years to educational services
• The educational process for children from 3-21 years

EARLY INTERVENTION SERVICES (0-3 YEARS)

Eligibility

An historic turning point in federal and state policy for disabled and developmentally vulnerable young children and their

187

families occurred in 1986 with the passage of **Public Law 99-457** (PL 99-457), the **Education of Handicapped Act Amendments.** PL 99-457 encouraged the development and implementation in each state of a "statewide, comprehensive, coordinated, multidisciplinary, interagency program of early intervention services for infants and toddlers and their families" (Part H of the law). It also provided incentives for states to serve all children who are disabled aged 3 through 5 years (Part B of the law).

PL 99-457 (Part H) applies to children 0-2 years. The majority of states have extended this coverage to include children up to 3 years old. PL 99-457 provides legal protections to children within one of two federally mandated categories and one optional category. The first category includes children who are delayed in at least 1 of 5 developmental areas, including cognition, physical skills (including vision and hearing), communication and psychosocial development, or self-help skills. The law specifies that individual states are to establish criteria to define what constitutes developmental delay. For example, New Jersey defines developmental delay as 33% delay in one developmental area, with the percentage calculated on the basis of chronological age, or 25% delay in two or more developmental areas with the percentage calculated on the basis of chronological age.

The second federally mandated category includes children who have a diagnosed physical or mental condition with a high probability of resulting in developmental delay (Mental Health Law Project, 1990). Examples of these conditions include fetal alcohol syndrome, seizure disorders, and chromosomal abnormalities such as **Down Syndrome.** The third category is optional and includes children who are at-risk for future developmental difficulties. This category may be used at the discretion of the state in which the child resides. At-risk conditions commonly are defined to include **very low birthweight** resulting from **prematurity** (such as Lisa), **respiratory distress, asphyxia,** and/or **intraventricular hemorrhage** (such as Frank) (See Chapter 1 for Lisa and Frank initial case histories.).

Legal Protection

Children who meet the eligibility requirements under PL 99-457 receive the following legal protections (National Early Childhood Technical Assistance System [NEC-TAS], 1989):

1. The right to consent to assessment, evaluation, and services;

2. The right to receive notice of their rights and of proposed actions by the early intervention system;
3. The right to review and correct records;
4. The right to require that private information be kept confidential; and
5. The right to have complaints resolved by an impartial decision-maker.

Care Providers

Children typically receive services by care providers as part of early intervention programs. Early intervention is designed to encourage normal developmental patterns, to prevent diagnosed conditions from becoming more disabling, and to improve the overall functioning of young children who have developmental delays or who are at-risk of becoming disabled. These services are provided by a core team of professionals who collaboratively evaluate, develop, and implement an individualized plan for the child and family. The core team of professionals in most early intervention programs consists of: early childhood special education, nursing, therapeutic recreation, social work, medicine, psychology, physical and occupational therapy, and speech-language pathology.

Early intervention is a team effort, required because the complexity of developmental disabilities precludes that no single discipline has sufficient knowledge to address all areas of care. Team efforts may be **multidisciplinary, interdisciplinary,** or **transdisciplinary**. Multidisciplinary teams are professionals performing related tasks independently of one another, a team by association only. This type of model is often seen in the medical field. Interdisciplinary teams are professionals performing related tasks independently, yet interacting to coordinate their efforts. The professionals constitute a team because they share information to reach a common goal. Goals and activities of one discipline support and complement those of other disciplines. Transdisciplinary teams are professionals performing related tasks interactively by sharing not only information but also roles. They constitute a team through their highly coordinated efforts to interact with one another (Meisels & Provence, 1989).

The Early Intervention Process: Referral to Service Delivery

Even though Lisa and Frank had different postnatal histories and family issues, the process of receiving early intervention services would be the same for each. All referred children go through the same steps in eligibility determination.

Referrals

A variety of sources offer referrals to early intervention programs, including, but not limited to, caregivers, physicians, neonatal follow-up programs, social service agencies, school districts, allied health professionals, and others in the medical community. Regulations require that on referral a **case manager** be assigned to the family. The case manager's role and function is to support and strengthen family functioning. Case managers are also responsible for coordinating the performance of evaluations and assessments, as well as linking the child's caregivers with community supports.

Evaluation

PL 99-457 requires that each child receive an evaluation performed by appropriately qualified personnel. The purpose of the evaluation is to determine the child's initial and continuing eligibility, including determination of the youngster's status in each of the five developmental areas determining PL99-457. Caregivers must give written consent for an evaluation. The early intervention program must ensure that the evaluation activities be conducted in a timely manner and be at least multidisciplinary.

PL 99-457 does not define children as isolated service recipients. Rather, children's needs are considered as embedded within the context of the overall family unit. Thus, early intervention is intended to address the individual needs of the child within the framework of the youngster's family. Because the child's family is central in early intervention efforts, it is important to assess the family as well as the child. The importance of assessing family strengths and needs is to empower caregivers by giving them the opportunity to state which factors in their family life might affect their ability to care for their special child. Examples of assessment instruments frequently used for this purpose include the *Family Needs Survey* (Bailey & Simonsson, 1985) and the *Family Needs Scale* (Dunst, Trivette, & Deal, 1988).

Lisa and Frank can serve to illustrate family assessments. The family of Lisa might have a profile:

Strengths: 1. Strong family support.
2. Ability to access community resources as needed.
3. Family intact.

Needs: 1. Family needs further information on prognosis in relationship to possible early medical complications.
2. Caregiver support involvement with other families of children with tracheostomies needed.

In contrast, the strengths and needs of Frank's family might be:

Strengths: 1. Mother electively attends rehabilitation program for substance abuse.
2. Mother and grandmother are supportive of one another in Frank's care.

Needs: 1. Financial support.
2. Medical training in tracheostomy care.
3. Assessment of medical and community resources for in-home care.
4. Information on developmental stimulation.
5. Community-based case management system to coordinate care and appointments.

Individualized Family Service Plan

Once the early intervention program has received a referral it has 45 days in which to complete the evaluation and assessment activities and to hold an **Individualized Family Service Plan (IFSP)** meeting. This 45-day timetable provides an important protection for children and their caregivers.

The purpose of the IFSP is to enable caregivers to make informed choices about the early intervention services they want for their children and themselves. The IFSP is developed through gathering, sharing, and exchanging information between caregivers and staff. Appendix 9-A contains a sample IFSP form.

The following information is included in the IFSP (NEC-TAS, 1989):

1. A statement of the child's levels of physical, cognitive, speech-language and psycho-social development, as well as self-help skills, based on acceptable objective criteria at the time of assessment;
2. A statement of the family's strengths and needs pertaining to enhancement of the child's development;
3. A statement of major outcomes expected to be achieved for the child and the family, including criteria, procedures, and timelines for determining the degree of progress toward achieving an outcome being made at given points and if and when modifications or revisions of outcomes or services might be necessary;

4. A statement of specific early intervention services necessary in meeting the unique needs of the child and the family, including the frequency, intensity, and the method of delivering services;
5. The projected dates for initiation of services and the anticipated duration of services;
6. The name of a case manager from the profession with skills most immediately relevant to the needs of the child and family as the staff responsible for the implementation of the plan and coordination with other agencies and persons; and
7. The steps to be taken for supporting the transition to services provided under PL 99-457 Part B, preschool services, to the extent such services are considered appropriate.

Appropriate Care

A major emphasis of the Part H program of PL 99-457 is that services provided must be "appropriate." Appropriate care includes (National Early Childhood Technical Assistance System [NEC-TAS], 1989):

1. Family training, counseling, and home visits;
2. Special instruction;
3. Developmental and rehabilitation therapies (speech pathology and audiology, occupational therapy, physical therapy);
4. Psychological services;
5. Case management services;
6. Medical services for diagnosis and evaluation;
7. Early identification, screening, and assessment services; and
8. Health services necessary to enable the child to benefit from other early intervention services.

Additionally, the law recognizes that the early intervention center may need to provide transportation to enable the child to receive early intervention services.

Lastly, PL 99-457 mandates that services are most appropriate when provided in the child's natural environment. This means that, when possible, services should be community-based, reducing the child's isolation from settings and activities in which children without special needs would participate. In the case of Lisa who was medically stable following **decannulation** at 14 months, the most appropriate setting would be a community-based early intervention program. In the case of Frank (who presented with ongoing medical complications), the most appropriate setting might be home-bound services. Depending on the service delivery model of the early intervention program, home-bound services could consist of one primary person (transdisciplinary approach) or several members of the treatment team (interdisciplinary approach) working in the home environment.

Transition to Preschool

Children must be placed in a preschool program by age 3 because at that age they no longer are eligible for early intervention services. To achieve a smooth transition between early intervention and preschool, the social worker on the early intervention team should notify the child's school district at least three months prior to the child's third birthday. At that time, the child study team from the district might establish a meeting with the child's family and the early intervention team to discuss the child's future educational and therapeutic needs.

SCHOOL-AGED POPULATION (AGES 3-21)

Eligibility

On November 29, 1975, President Gerald Ford signed **The Education for All Handicapped Children Act (PL 94-142)**. This federal law mandated the provision of free, appropriate education to all children with handicaps aged 3 through 21 years, established evaluation and assessment policies, guaranteeing the right to due process of law, and established a process for financial support of educational services. The law was amended in 1990 to include more populations of children as eligible for special education and related services, authorized and expanded a number of discretionary programs, and mandated transition services and assistive technology services in a child's education program.

Legal Protection

PL 94-142 mandates that all children with handicaps have the legal right to receive a free and appropriate education. These rights include entitlement to the following services (Lovitt, 1988; Administration on Developmental Disabilities, 1988):

1. A thorough assessment in a nondiscriminatory manner to determine the nature and degree of specific disability, with no single measurement being the sole criterion for evaluation;
2. A free education appropriately tailored to meet the individual needs of the child;

3. Placement in the "least restrictive environment" with emphasis on placing children who are disabled with typical children; and

4. The provision of supplementary aid and services to help ensure a program success for each child.

The Education Process: Referral to Service Delivery

The referral process begins when there is a concern about the child's performance in the classroom, home, or other setting. The purpose of the referral is to formally indicate that a particular child is not performing as well as peers. The referral allows for a request of assistance in investigating if a problem exists and, if so, the nature of the problem. Referrals can be generated by any number of individuals, including, but not limited to caregivers, teachers, school principals, social service agencies, or other individuals involved with the child.

The two most common referrals are from regular teachers and caregivers. Teacher-initiated referrals usually originate with a classroom teacher with concerns about the child's academic performance or behavior. Common reasons for referral include inability to complete daily work assignments, poor attention span, difficulty with peer relationships, and below-grade-level performance. Although referrals are usually initiated by the classroom teacher, caregivers may also express their concerns, thereby initiating the referral process.

Evaluation

Once a referral has been initiated, there are three questions that should be asked:

1. Is there a school performance problem?
2. Is the problem related to a handicapping condition?
3. What are the student's educational needs?

The educational assessment of students who are handicapped is the systematic process of gathering educational information relevant to the above three questions and making legal decisions about the provision of special services. Procedural safeguards in assessment include the notification and consent of caregivers and the student in selection of special education and tests. Decisions based on the evaluation process are interpreted legally as a change of status in the student's school program.

There are two principle types of evaluations: screenings and educational assessments. Screenings are performed to identify those students who may have a severe learning disability. Screening procedures should be efficient, time-effective and reliable. During the screening, the student's instructional environment at that time is examined and alternative strategies are explored to better accommodate academic and behavioral needs.

The educational assessment is performed to determine (1) if the child is eligible to receive special education, and (2) if school performance problems are related to a handicapping condition. In general, educational assessments are administered in the areas of school achievement, social skill development, intelligence, and related areas.

For both screenings and educational assessments, PL 94-142 stipulates that the following procedural safeguards are to be followed (Lovitt, 1988):

1. Tests and other evaluation materials must be provided and administered in the child's native language or other mode of communication, unless it is not feasible to do so;
2. Tests and other evaluation materials must have been validated for the purpose for which they are used;
3. Tests and other evaluation materials must be administered by trained personnel in conformance with the instructions provided by the test developer-publisher;
4. Tests and other evaluation materials must assess specific areas of educational need, not simply general intelligence measures;
5. Tests must be selected and administered to best ensure that a child with impaired sensory, manual, or speaking skills, will be tested for accurate reflection of the child's aptitude or achievement level or whatever other factor the test purports to measure, rather than a reflection of the child's impaired sensory, manual, or speaking skills;
6. No single procedure should be used as the sole criterion for determining an appropriate educational program for the child;
7. The evaluation should be made by a multidisciplinary team or group of persons, including at least one teacher or other specialist with knowledge in the area of the suspected disability; and
8. The child should be assessed in all areas related to the suspected disability, including, where appropriate, health, vision, hearing, social and emotional status, general intelligence, academic performance, communicative status, and motor abilities.

Individualized Educational Plan (IEP)

The educational assessment is used in program planning to develop the **Individualized Education Plan (IEP)**. An IEP is a written statement for a child who is handicapped describing the educational objectives for that child and the special services to be provided. Stated informally, the IEP should describe how the child was assessed, what and how the child should be taught, where the teaching will take place and by whom, and how to tell if the program is working and the child is learning. More formally, the IEP must contain the following (Lovitt, 1988):

1. A statement of the child's levels of educational performance at the time of assessment;
2. A statement of annual goals, including short-term instructional objectives;
3. A statement of specific special education and related services to be provided to the child, and the extent to which the child will be able to participate in regular educational programs;
4. The projected dates for initiation of services and the anticipated duration of the services; and
5. The appropriate objective criteria and evaluation procedures, and schedules for determining on at least an annual basis if the short-term instructional objectives are being achieved.

At least three people must be involved in developing the IEP: (a) a representative of the public agency who is qualified to provide or supervise the provision of special education; (b) the child's teacher and (c) the child (when appropriate) and one or both of the child's legal guardians. The IEP must be in effect before special education and related services are provided to a child and be implemented as soon as possible following the meeting.

Appropriate Care

Children with tracheostomies receive services within a variety of education models, each of which offers both advantages and disadvantages (Mercer, 1987).

The preferred educational model is the exclusive placement in a typical classroom. The advantage of this model is that it prevents labeling and stigmatization. Additionally, it is the least restrictive of settings and affords extensive opportunities for the child to interact with children without disabilities. The disadvantage of the model is that it is only appropriate for children with milder disabilities, because instruction in regular classrooms is rarely geared for the child with developmental problems. Further, typical classes often contain a large number of children, which reduces opportunities for individualized instruction and may pose severe challenges for children with attention difficulties. Lastly, teachers in regular classes typically do not have the specialized training required to provide instruction to children with disabilities.

The most commonly encountered model for children with developmental disabilities involves the use of a resource teacher. Within this model, the child spends a portion of the school day (typically, from 45 minutes to 1 hour) with a resource teacher in a resource room. Advantages of this model are that it reduces stigmatization because the child spends the majority of time in a typical classroom. An additional important advantage is that this model provides the child an opportunity to receive specialized instruction and individual attention in problem areas. An important disadvantage of this model is that, because of limited amount of available time with the resource teacher, it is not appropriate for a child with severe developmental handicaps.

Children with the more severe developmental disabilities might be provided services in one of three education models: **special classes, special day schools,** and **residential schools.** Within the special class model, a child spends the majority of the school day in a special education class. An advantage of such a setting is that it is the least restrictive setting for children with more severe developmental difficulties, it provides individual or small group instruction, and it offers the services of a teacher specially trained to meet the needs of children with developmental difficulties. Possible disadvantages of this model are that it segregates children with disabilities from other children and that placements in such settings are usually permanent, sometimes even when the child's condition improves.

The special day school model of education is a model of education in which children spend entire school days in special schools. Major advantages of the special day school model are that all educational services are centralized, the environment is specially developed to meet the child's needs, and the child is allowed to remain in the home and community. The major disadvantages of the model are that it is self-contained, the child has no interactions with children without disabilities, and such schools can sometimes be expensive.

The last major model of education is the residential school. In this model, children live in special schools. The advantage of this model is that children can efficiently receive occupational training and special diet, as well as necessary medical treatment. These schools also provide children with disabilities the opportunity to become involved in all aspects of typical school life. The major disadvantages of this model are that it is segregated, is often financially expensive, and few children who are enrolled in residential schools later return to more mainstream educational settings.

CONCLUSIONS

The members of the health care team need to be knowledgeable about their patients' legal right to receive education services to best help plan for these children's future and to counsel the child's caregivers. Services for children with developmental and physical disabilities and their families have improved substantially in the past 25 years. Federal legislation has played an integral part in this improvement through the creation of policies, procedures, and funding that enable infants and children with handicaps to receive services and educational programs to meet their needs. Educational planning for special needs children will inevitably continue to undergo change as new federal legislation is introduced and individual states interpret existing and new federal guidelines. Those working with such youngsters need to continually be alert to future developments.

REFERENCES

Administration on Developmental Disabilities (1988). *Mapping the future for children with special needs: P.L. 99-457.* Iowa City: University of Iowa Press.
Bailey, D., & Simonsson, R. (1985). *Family needs survey.* Chapel Hill: The University of North Carolina at Chapel Hill.
Dunst, C., Trivette, C., & Deal, A. (1988). *Enabling and empowering families: Principles and guidelines for practice.* Cambridge, Brookline Books.
Jordon, J., Gallagher, J., Hutinger, P. Karnes, M. (1988). *Early childhood special education: Birth to three.* Reston, VA: Council for Exceptional Children.
Lovitt, T. (1988). *Writing and implementing an IEP: A step-by-step plan.* Belmont, CA: Fearson Education.
Meisels, S., & Provence, S. (1989). *Screening and assessment: Guidelines for identifying young disabled and developmentally vulnerable children and their families.* Washington, DC: National Center for Clinical Infant Programs.
Mental Health Law Project. (1990). *Early intervention advocacy network: Guide to Part H law and regulations.* Washington, DC.: Mental Health Law Project.
Mercer, C (1987). *Students with learning disabilities* (3rd ed.). Columbus, OH: Merrill.

McGongigel, M., Kaufmann, R., & Johnson, B. (Eds.). (1991). *National Early Childhood Technical Assistance System (NEC-TAS): Guidelines and recommended practices for the individualized family service plan* (2nd ed.). Chapel Hill, NC: National Early Childhood Technical Assistance System.

U. S. Department of Education, Office of Special Education and Rehabilitative Services. (1991). Thirteenth annual report to Congress on the Implementation of the Individuals with Disabilities Act. Washington, DC.

APPENDIX 9-A

Sample Form of an Individualized Family Service Plan

1. Background Information

Child's Name: _____

Date of Birth: _____

Referral Source: _____

Caregiver(s)/Guardian(s) Name: _____

Address: _____

_____

Telephone (days): _____

Telephone (evenings): _____

Consent for Evaluation: _____

Date of Evaluation: _____

School District: _____

Case Manager: _____

Case Manager (telephone) _____

2. Statement of Eligibility*

_____ is eligible for Early
Intervention services because:

_____ .

* Each state has its own guidelines for admission to an early intervention program.

IFSP TEAM
Caregiver/Guardian Signature   Date

_____

_____

_____

Professional Personnel Signature Date

_____
_____
_____
_____

3. Current Status

HEALTH STATUS:

SOCIAL SUMMARY:

FAMILY STRENGTHS AND NEEDS:

DEVELOPMENTAL AREAS:
    Physical: _____
    Adaptive: _____
    Sensory: _____
    Communication: _____
    Social-Emotional: _____

DIAGNOSTIC TOOLS USED FOR EVALUATION/ASSESSMENT:
    Physical: _____
    Adaptive: _____
    Sensory: _____
    Communication: _____
    Social-Emotional: _____

4. Services to be Provided
Type of Service(s): _____
Frequency: _____
Intensity: _____
Location: _____

5. Recommendations for Further Services and Evaluations

_____
_____
_____
_____

10

The Social Worker's Role With the Family

Linda Hock-Long, Symme W. Trachtenberg, and Dolores Vorters

INTRODUCTION

This chapter describes the provision of social work services to the family whose child requires technological assistance. The major focus is on helping families successfully manage home care. The following topics are addressed:

- Initial assessment of the family
- Impact of the hospitalization on the family
- Decision making for home care
- Transition to home
- Care in the home

IN THE HOSPITAL

The hospitalization of a child who has serious medical problems and requires life-supporting technology is, undoubtedly, one of the most stressful events a family will ever face. Because of the many difficulties that arise for families who have children needing **long-term tracheostomies** or **ventilator assistance,** social work staff should be available to them as early as possible in the hospitalization to provide counseling, advocacy, and case management services.

One of the social worker's first goals on meeting a family is to begin to develop a supportive, trusting relationship with them. The social worker, hopefully, achieves this goal by expressing an interest in all family members and appearing knowledgeable of specific medical, emotional, and financial issues encountered by families of children requiring technological assistance. The social worker can also serve to facilitate the family-hospital staff relationship. By sharing pertinent information with appropriate staff, the social worker can help them to more fully understand the family and work as effectively as possible with them.

Initial Assessment

An initial psychosocial assessment provides the social worker with an organized mechanism for gathering information to help in evaluating a family's values, strengths, and limitations in relation to their child's medical problems and prognosis. Such an instrument is a guide to identify areas that will need to be addressed to assist the family in managing the challenges of hospitalization and discharge planning.

The initial psychosocial assessment should contain demographic information for each caregiver, including name, marital status, date of birth, address, home telephone number, highest educational level attained, occupation; employer, work telephone number, religious preference, and type of medical care coverage. Information on siblings should list their dates of birth and any special needs they might have. The initial assessment should also list any other persons composing the household and their relation to the hospitalized child, and the names of persons to contact if caregivers cannot be reached in an emergency. It is also important to learn if there are any custody/guardianship issues that need to be considered and if there is any type of active community agency involvement.

In addition to providing background information, the initial assessment should explore the following to develop an understanding of and appreciation for the individual family:

1. Relevant family history, such as recent caregiver illness, history of caregiver learning difficulties
2. Family's understanding of why current services are being provided
3. Family's satisfaction level with services
4. Family's understanding of child's medical and developmental problems

5. Family's description of the child, for example functional changes that have resulted from the medical problems, perceptions about the child's personality and temperament style
6. Family's perception of their own reactions to their child's illness and ability to manage current situation
7. Family's past experience with illness and loss
8. Family's discharge expectations
9. Identification of additional stresses, for example developmental problems of another child in the family, recent job loss
10. Quality and reliability of support systems
11. Family's financial status, including current source of medical benefits

Social Work Services

It is widely agreed that during acute periods in the hospitalization of the child who has a **tracheostomy** or is ventilator-assisted, families wrestle with feelings of shock, grief, and sadness. They must adjust to the severity of the medical issues and, in some cases, to the possibility that their child may die. People in crisis react in a variety of ways. Some families may hover over their child's bed or turn to prayer—others leave the hospital, not wanting to return until a complete recovery has been made. Others may react by expressing anger or criticism toward hospital staff. Members of the same family might have disparate ways of coping and, therefore, be unable to support one another. The social worker can be instrumental in helping the family deal with the stress of the hospitalization and understand each other's behavior. In addition, the social worker can assist the other support staff in recognizing the family's coping behaviors.

During hospitalization, it is of utmost importance for families to stay actively involved with their child. This can be especially challenging if the hospital stay is lengthy, the hospital is located at a distance, there are other children at home, or caregivers are employed. With multiple professional caretakers, caregivers may sometimes feel superfluous or inadequate in caring for their child. Caregivers may also be disturbed by the sight of their child's tracheostomy, ventilator, and other sophisticated, unfamiliar medical equipment. All these factors may heighten caregiver feelings of loss of control and disrupt the bonding/attachment process (Scharer & Dixon, 1989).

Social workers can play a significant role in facilitating family involvement in the hospital. They can educate families about the hospital, staff functions, and hierarchies that might affect them. The social worker can discuss the importance of the family to the hospitalized child and encourage their participation in the child's daily routine. If a family is apprehensive about performing tracheostomy or ventilator care, the social worker can attempt to help them discover more comfortable ways of interacting—such as rocking a baby, reading to an older child, and so on. Such interventions can be beneficial in several ways. First, with an increased understanding of the hospital system and the crucial role of the family, caregivers may be empowered to communicate more effectively with staff and participate more fully in their child's care. Also, by working together on these issues, the relationship between the family and social worker may be strengthened. These experiences will allow the family to better appreciate that the social worker is a member of the hospital team to whom they can turn when concerns arise.

Many families are uncomfortable talking with members of the hospital staff. For some, the hospital environment seems like a foreign land where they have little understanding of the language or customs. Other families may not be able to formulate questions or recognize that their input is helpful to the staff. In such instances, the social worker can work to enhance caregiver-staff communication. By assisting caregivers in preparing questions, arranging meetings, and encouraging an open dialogue, the social worker can help both caregivers and staff become more effective communicators. It is advisable to hold formal caregiver-staff meetings periodically throughout the hospitalization of a child requiring technological assistance. These meetings should be scheduled routinely so that problems can be managed and short- and long-term goals can be achieved as efficiently as possible. Generally, it is helpful to hold meetings as follows: at the time of admission, at intervals when there is new information or the family has diagnostic or prognostic questions, when there is a significant change in the child's status, and throughout the discharge planning process.

In addition to helping with emotional and adjustment issues, the social worker is available to help caregivers address practical problems. For example, to be able to visit at the hospital, some caregivers may need to find baby-sitting services for their other children. By discussing possible alternatives with the caregivers, the social worker can help them define their support system, needs for which they may have to rely on community services, and how they can advocate for themselves. Through the process of working on practical problems, caregivers can learn to become more capable advocates—a skill that will serve them well if they decide to take their child home from the hospital (Dunst, Trivette, Davis, & Cornwell, 1988).

Connecting a family with an appropriate support group is another service that can be of value. Some hospitals have volunteer support groups often organized by caregivers whose children have or have had special medical needs. Such "trained" caregivers may provide insightful information, support, and empathetic hospital coping strategies. Additionally, the social worker can educate families about publications and other community resources that might be useful. Appendix 10-A provides suggested readings for health care providers and caregivers on these and related topics.

DISCHARGE PLANNING

Social workers play an integral role in planning for the discharge of the child who has a tracheostomy or requires mechanical ventilation. They work in conjunction with the family and other members of the health care team to determine if home care is an appropriate choice, secure funding, select home care service providers, and locate community services that may be of assistance. Successful discharge of a child who is technologically assisted to the home ultimately depends on the capacity of the family, the child's medical status, and the level of care required. The two most critical factors contributing to the successful outcome of community-based care are adequate funding and self-confident, well-trained families. If the possibility of home care is to become a reality, careful planning and close teamwork are essential.

The process of discharge planning often begins informally. For example, families may notice another child being prepared for care outside of the hospital and inquire about home care. Discharge possibilities might also be discussed during conversations caregivers have with the physician, nurse, social worker, therapist, or other hospital staff member. Regardless of how the topic of home care originates, it needs to be dealt with thoughtfully, as caring in a home for a child with a tracheostomy or ventilator represents a significant commitment for all involved. The critical difference in home care of the child who has a tracheostomy or is ventilator assisted and the child who is dependent on any other technology is the absolute necessity of constant and vigilant observation.

It must be recognized that, in some situations, home care is not an option (Hochstadt, Neil, & Yost, 1989; Trachtenberg, 1992). Even though children may be medically stable, discharge to their biologic families may not be feasible for such reasons as inadequate supports for the caregivers, inability of the family to learn care, unwillingness to learn care, and attachment issues. Social work involvement in these cases is essential. Through their understanding of community resources, the social worker can work with the health care team, family, and child welfare agency to determine appropriate alternatives—such as continued hospitalization, medical foster care, or a skilled nursing facility. The social worker can then investigate the alternatives, provide support and counseling to the family, and consult with potential providers of community services.

PLANNING FOR HOME CARE

Home care for children who are medically stable and require long-term tracheostomies and mechanical ventilatory assistance has become an increasingly popular alternative to hospitalization since the early 1980s. There is now general consensus that discharging children to a home setting is developmentally, medically, and economically preferable to long-term hospitalization (Fields, 1982; Gillis et al., 1989; Hazlett, 1989). Although the advantages of home care are certainly significant, it is also recognized that transitioning a child from hospital to home is a challenging undertaking for all involved (Schreiner, Donar, & Kettrick, 1987; Quint, Chesterman, Crain, Winkleby, & Boyce, 1990). The complex care of the child who requires technological assistance, the demands placed on the family, and the frequent lack of adequate funding for home care services often make discharge planning difficult. Social work education and training, which includes development of clinical skills and knowledge of public and private service systems, prepares the social worker to work with the family that has a child with chronic health problems.

The following areas must be carefully addressed in planning for care at home. It is important that the social worker is aware of progress in all areas to best advocate for the caregiver and child, especially if the social worker is functioning as the case manager.

Family Preparation

One of the primary tasks of the social worker is to assist families in planning for their child's discharge. It is understood that families vary in their ability to meet children's care needs, and the social worker can be helpful in devising individualized home care preparation strategies. For example, some families may master the technical aspects of tracheostomy and ventilator care, but find the care to be emotionally difficult to perform, while others may experience difficulty in achieving competency in the intricacies of the home procedures (Lynch, 1990). To determine if a family is ready to take their child home, the social worker should assist them in deciding if they will be able to provide the required level of supervision and care. It may be helpful to assess stress factors that could affect a family's readiness by exploring areas such as those presented in Table 10-1.

As indicated, for a child who is technology-assisted to go home, the caregiver or caretaker must be thoroughly trained in all aspects of care. Caregivers must understand their child's illness and achieve independence with all tracheostomy and ventilator procedures. In addition, if the child requires additional specialized care—such as gastrostomy tube feedings, range of motion exercises—competency in these areas must also be achieved. It is necessary for at least two caregivers to be completely trained and capable of caring for the child by themselves. If possible, it is advisable to have a third trained caregiver available. Any designated caregiver must understand the level of responsibility to be assumed in caring for a child with a tracheostomy or ventilator.

Home care nursing is not typically provided 24 hours per day. Therefore, families need to recognize that they will sometimes be alone with their child. In an effort to increase caretakers' proficiency and confidence, it is important to include an opportunity for them to have complete care responsibility as part of their home care training. This can be done in the hospital or at home, if a child is able to have a therapeutic pass before discharge.

TABLE 10-1. Common stress factors of home care on families.

NUMBER	STRESS FACTORS
1.	Fear of child's death at home
2.	Fatigue
3.	Financial worries
4.	Impact on other family members
5.	Decreased social mobility
6.	Inability to explore employment opportunities because of dependence on specific job-related insurance
7.	Worry regarding possibility that medical supplies will not be delivered in a timely fashion
8.	Lack of privacy in home because of presence of home health care staff
9.	Concerns about child's long-term medical and developmental prognosis

Counseling during the discharge planning process often focuses on family adjustment themes. Concerns such as fear about the future or guilt caregivers may have about their perceived contribution to their child's medical and/or developmental problems need to be identified and openly addressed. Through this process, caregivers can often come to "own" these feelings, try to understand them, and emotionally move on. The social worker should also address the reactions of the child's siblings and other significant family members. When appropriate, counseling and mental health intervention are offered.

Home Care Costs and Funding

Home care is a costly service presenting a prohibitive burden for the majority of families. The resources available to make the transition from hospital to home possible include: commercial insurers, health maintenance organizations, Medicaid, and Medicaid waiver programs.

Securing funding for home care is often contingent on demonstrating that it is a cost-effective alternative to institutional care. The costs of an entire home care package (equipment, supplies, nursing, rehabilitation services, and so on) need to be compared to in-patient costs. Showing that home care actually results in a savings encourages many third-party payers to authorize funding.

Personal financial resources should be examined by the family before taking home a child who is technology-assisted. The utility bills will undoubtedly increase because of electrical equipment required. Telephone bills may also increase if the physician or hospital is at a distance from the home. All of the utility companies must be aware that a child on life support is present in the home and requires uninterrupted service. The caregivers should be encouraged to seek out assistance with their utility bills, such as arranging reasonable payment plans with the utilities. Most public utility companies are very willing to work with the family in these special circumstances.

It is extremely important that the family comprehends the benefits and limitations of their health care coverage. Third-party payer approval for home care should be obtained and verified while the child is still in the hospital or long-term care facility. An extensive letter of medical necessity is often required by insurers. Such a letter explains the child's diagnosis and history, rationale for nursing and/or rehabilitation therapies, equipment required in the home, and an estimate of the length of time the care may be necessary.

If benefits do not exist for home care, efforts to obtain an out-of-benefit exception should be made. Areas to focus on include converting in-patient hospital days to home care days and looking at in-patient costs versus home care costs to demonstrate to an insurance group the financial benefits of home care. Legal advice can be sought through patient advocacy groups familiar with home care law to guide families through this process. The family should also be encouraged to employ their local political resources to support the home care plan.

State model waiver programs may be an option if insurance has been exhausted or a child is covered under Medicaid. Model waiver programs vary from state to state, and the social worker should be knowledgeable about the possibility of coverage under this plan (Murray, 1989). All model waiver programs include an extensive application process that examines available health insurance and a physician's statement of diagnosis(es), related medical problems, and care needs. This process is time-consuming and should be explored well in advance of an anticipated discharge or exhaustion of insurance benefits.

Home Care Services

When discharge of a child who is technology-assisted is anticipated, considerable thought should be given to the choice of home care provider agencies. The social worker and other hospital staff may be familiar with a number of home care agencies and the services provided. Some agencies offer multiple services—for example, nursing, social work, infusion support, and respiratory and rehabilitation therapies—while others supply a single service. Families should be given the names of contact persons with home care providers. Independently or in conjunction with hospital personnel, the family can interview representatives of various companies and determine which seems most appropriate. With managed care plans, the family may not have a choice of provider agency. (Families seem most satisfied when they have the opportunity to choose their home care provider[s].)

Some insurers may offer the family the option to independently hire staff. This may be a cost-saving option, but requires that the family interview, screen, hire, schedule and terminate, when necessary, the nurses or aides. Such a system can be workable if the family is able to access skilled caregivers. However, as the availability of staff can fluctuate, this may be a difficult proposition over time.

When choosing a nursing agency, part of the interviewing process should include an examination of the professional backgrounds and expertise of the staff. Companies supplying respiratory services and rehabilitation therapists should likewise be interviewed and screened. Ideally, home care staff will have pediatric training and experience.

Rehabilitation therapies are needed by many children requiring tracheostomies and ventilator assistance at home. Often insurance coverage for speech, occupational, and physical therapy is limited. Thus, it is extremely important that the social worker be aware of early intervention, special preschool, and special educational services that are available in the community. Many programs are developing the capacity to serve children who are medically fragile and have staff available to meet the needs of the child who requires technological assistance.

Social work services should be available to all children at home with tracheostomies and mechanical ventilation. These services may be provided by the hospital-based social worker or the home care agency social worker, depending on the needs of the family and the availability of services. Every family, no matter how well prepared, experiences stress with the changes in their home. It can be very therapeutic for the caregivers and/or the child to have access to a professional who understands the situation, but does not provide direct care. As during the hospitalization, the social worker can offer a range of services including counseling, advocacy, case management, referral, and support.

In addition to providing service to the family and child, the social worker can be of assistance to other home care staff. Working in the home can be an intense experience. It is, therefore, helpful for staff to communicate with one another. Home care staff are more isolated than those working in the hospital, and the social worker can facilitate communication and team-building activities. Such facilitation enhances greatest satisfaction for all involved.

Home Preparation

The home of the child who is technology-assisted must be assessed to assure that care at the site is manageable and safe. This includes looking at basic utility services such as heat, electricity, telephone, and water. The availability of these resources at the required levels must be assured, as the patient's care would be affected with service disruption. Before the child leaves the hospital, the utility companies must be notified in writing of a patient's dependence on life support for the child's placement on a service priority list. Local fire, police, and/or emergency services should also be notified of a patient dependent on life-support equipment to alert them to the need for appropriate rescue and electrical generator equipment in emergencies.

The patient's care environment (room) requires adequate electrical outlets, good ventilation, and enough space for equipment and access by caregivers. It is helpful to have the child's bed, equipment and disposable supplies delivered and set up before the youngster arrives from the hospital. All equipment should be tested and ready to run before the commencement of home care.

Careful planning for emergencies is imperative. For example, it is advisable to have a written emergency plan close to the telephone and the care area. This plan should include: the patient's name, address, and telephone number; the emergency service number; the physician's number; and directions to the child's home. Another helpful strategy is to provide the emergency service and the nearest hospital with an up-to-date copy of the child's medical summary before hospital discharge.

HOME CARE

The effect of a child in the home with a tracheostomy on family life cannot be overestimated, especially if the child also receives ventilator assistance (Wegener & Aday, 1989). Quint et al. (1990) report on a survey of 18 Northern California families. All but one were intact, two-caregiver households. Neurologic conditions were the predominant underlying diagnoses, with only one child having a primary pulmonary problem; however, 83% had additional medical problems. Equipment problems or difficulty with vendors occurred up to 20 times for 2/3 of the families. Seventy-two percent had in-home nursing care for more than 9 hours per day. Although 71% felt this was an invasion of privacy, most emphasized their reliance on the care. Of particular note is that the perceived stress of the primary caregiver increased over time.

Family-Home Care Staff Relationships

Imagine having a house guest 8, 16, or 24 hours a day, 7 days a week. Consider the restrictions of having a professional in the home observing almost everything you do. Think about having to seek out privacy to hold a family discussion. These are some of the situations that often arise when a child with a tracheostomy or ventilator is cared for at home. The family must recognize that previous typical routines will be affected by the presence of home care staff.

Transitioning from the "known" environment of the hospital to the "unknown" of the home and home care staff can be stressful for the caregivers, the child, and other family members. Stress can lead to an initial interpersonal awkwardness—trust takes time to develop, particularly in managing life-supporting care. This process can be assisted by encouraging open communication between the family and staff.

A challenging and emerging issue in home care involves professional boundaries. For example, if a home care staff person is always available and willing to give up personal time to assist a family, overdependence may develop. This can lead to family members expecting "solutions" from the professional whenever issues arise. The professional may then lose objectivity and the family may lose confidence in their own skills. In the end, this pattern will defeat one of the primary goals of home care, family independence. Such an outcome can be avoided by educating home care staff and families as part of the discharge planning process. The social worker is in a key position to be able to anticipate such dilemmas and intervene if problems should begin to develop at home.

Impact On Family

As indicated in Quint et al.'s study (1990), caring for a child who is technology-assisted at home has great impact on the family. In addition to traditional caregiver activities, caregivers need to develop skills as their child's care manager, nurse, and insurance expert.

During discharge planning, caregivers frequently do not consider the repercussions on their personal lives of having their technology-assisted child at home. Every caregiver needs some time for themselves, and considerable planning may be required in arranging for this. Some insurers will approve an increase in nursing hours to 24 hours a day to allow for respite. If 24-hour coverage is not permitted, the other professional caregivers could, perhaps, care for the child when a nurse is not there.

The siblings' needs may or may not be better met through home care. It should be explained that discharge to home does not necessarily mean that their brother or sister is "better." In fact, in some families, the child assisted by technology can become more of a focus than anticipated before discharge. Caregivers and home care staff need to be cognizant of all of the needs of the individual children in the family and attempt to find ways to meet various requirements. For example, the individual sibling's age, relationship with the caregivers and with the child who is technology-assisted will all influence a sibling's adaptation. The effect on siblings in the same family can vary—for example, some may become jealous of the care given by the nurses and caregivers, others attempt to assist with care, and some are appreciative that they have greater access to their caregivers who no longer make lengthy hospital visits. The social worker can be helpful to caregivers and staff in determining ways to incorporate siblings into the new milieu created by home care. If problems should occur, the social worker can also provide intervention options.

CASE STUDIES

Despite the many obstacles to providing home care, many families successfully undertake this challenge. Lisa and Frank (see introductory case histories in Chapter 1) represent two degrees of success in provision of home care services.

Lisa

As described in Chapter 1, Lisa was born at 32 weeks, weighing approximately 2,000 g. Lisa required ventilatory assistance at 3 months because of **bronchopulmonary dysplasia (BPD)**. Lisa's family consisted of her natural mother and father, Lisa's twin sister, and an older brother. Lisa's family participated in her care in the hospital. Her father was the more hesitant of the two caregivers in providing Lisa's care. Lisa's brother, Sam, was 6 when she was born. He visited her in the hospital 1-2 times per month, with his visits increasing as her discharge date approached.

Lisa's family lived in a row home in a working-class neighborhood, located approximately 30 minutes by car from the pediatric hospital where Lisa was followed by a pulmonologist. Lisa had a local pediatrician for routine issues, but her family felt more comfortable with the hospital pulmonologist assuming the major role in Lisa's medical care. Lisa's father worked 12 hours daily, usually 6 days a week. Lisa's father's family lived out of state, and her mother's family lived nearby.

Medical coverage for Lisa was originally provided through a commercial health insurance company. However, as her benefits were exhausted by the time she was ready to go home, application was made to the state model waiver program. Fortunately, Lisa was accepted into one of the program slots, and her home care needs were funded through this source. When Lisa was first discharged from the hospital, nursing care was provided for 24 hours per day for a 2-week period. After that, nursing coverage was approved for 16 hours per day. The group of nurses caring for Lisa remained relatively stable.

Rehabilitation services were provided for 60 days following hospital discharge. Before these services expired, referrals were made to a local, state-funded early intervention program, which could not provide therapists for direct care. An early education specialist, with consultation from a speech-language pathologist and physical therapist saw Lisa for home-bound early intervention. A social worker was available through the agency providing nursing care. On an average of 1-2 times per month a nurse had to cancel a shift and Lisa's caregivers then had responsibility for 16 hours of Lisa's care. Lisa's father did not feel comfortable caring for her without the direct assistance of another person, and her mother, therefore, needed to be available if a nurse was not.

Lisa's brother, Sam, had been under the impression that Lisa would be "all better" when she came home. Even though his caregivers, teacher, and hospital staff tried to prepare him for what it would be like with Lisa at home, it was not until she actually arrived that he realized she would continue to require special care.

Even though Lisa's family believed the decision to have Lisa at home while still ventilator-assisted was the best for their family, they found that they needed some relief from the demands of her care. After Lisa had been home for several months, her caregivers attempted to alleviate some of the stress by planning a 3-day vacation with Sam and Lisa's twin to a small resort. They obtained approval from the model waiver program for 24-hours-a-day service while away. Lisa's maternal grandmother agreed to stay at the house, but was unable to handle Lisa's total care. It was arranged that if the grandmother should become ill, Lisa's aunt—who lived across town, had a family, and worked outside the home full time—would take her place. Lisa's caregivers were planning to leave written instructions providing both Lisa's grandmother and aunt permission for Lisa's medical treatment, should a problem develop. Unfortunately, Lisa developed pneumonia several days before the vacation was to begin and the trip was canceled.

Home care for Lisa was discontinued when she was weaned from the ventilator and decannulated at 14 months of age.

Frank

As indicated in Chapter 1, Frank's mother was an occasional drug user when pregnant. He was born prematurely and had a stormy course the first several months. Frank was weaned from the ventilator at 10 months. His mother missed many training sessions on tracheostomy care at the hospital, and because of this, Frank was unable to be discharged until 15 months of age.

Frank lived with his mother and maternal grandmother in a two-story house. Frank's mother worked occasionally and his grandmother was retired. Frank's father had left the family before the child's birth and maintained only minimal contact—he visited Frank twice during the 15-month hospitalization. Frank's mother's extended family lived nearby. Although they were afraid to learn tracheostomy care, they did provide emotional support.

Frank received 8 hours of nursing care daily for the first week he was home. Frank's medical expenses were covered by his state's Medicaid program, which did not provide for shift nursing. After the first week, he was approved to have weekly nursing visits to monitor his progress.

One of the major stresses for Frank's mother and grandmother was the lack of other skilled caretakers. Several months after going home, Frank was admitted to the hospital due to tracheitis. During this hospitalization, his grandmother shared that his mother had again become involved with drugs. This information coincided with concerns about the care his mother was providing that had been raised by the respiratory equipment supplier staff.

Although Frank's mother visited him regularly in the hospital, she was able to admit to the social worker that she felt overwhelmed by the level of care he required at home. She acknowledged that she had an addiction problem and accepted a referral to an out-patient rehabilitation program. Because of these developments, it was necessary for Frank to remain in the hospital until another caretaker was identified and training was completed. As part of the discharge planning, the social worker was able to help the mother and maternal grandmother by arranging for in-home social service supports that included a social worker who provided counseling and a homemaker who assisted with medical appointments and budgeting issues. In addition, preparations were made for Frank to attend an early intervention program for medically fragile children two mornings a week. The hospital social worker remained as a liaison between the team at the hospital and the involved community services. Frank required no additional hospitalizations and was successfully decannulated at 30 months of age.

CONCLUSIONS

Medical advances of the past 10-15 years have made it possible for children to survive previously fatal neonatal medical conditions.

These children now pose challenges to their families, the medical community, and society. Because the care demands of the child who requires a tracheostomy or mechanical ventilation are great, no one person, or single discipline, alone can provide all the necessary care.

The concept of the Circle of Care, which is often used in designing and implementing HIV/AIDS services, represents the joining of separate individuals and organizations to surround and support a patient and family. The Circle of Care model is applicable in the situation of the child who receives technological assistance and the youngster's family. The social worker, as a member of the Circle of Care for this population, plays a vital role in helping the child, family, and other involved professionals. This chapter has described the contribution of the social worker during hospitalization and in home care. The greatest attention has been given to home care issues, because of the many challenges entailed in providing such services.

REFERENCES

Dunst, J., Trivette, C., Davis, M., & Cornwell, J. (1988). Enabling and empowering families of children with health impairments. *Children's Health Care, 17,* 71-81.

Fields, G. (1982). Social implications of long-term illness in children. In J. Downey & N. Low (Eds.), *The child with disabling illness: Principles of rehabilitation.* (pp. 595-610). New York: Raven Press.

Gillis, J., Tibballs, J., McEniery, J., Heavens, J., Hutchins, P., Kilham, H., & Henning, R. (1989). Ventilator dependent children. *The Medical Journal of Australia, 150,* 10-14.

Hazlett, D. (1989). A study of pediatric home ventilator management: Medical, psychosocial and financial aspects. *Journal of Pediatric Nursing, 4,* 284-293.

Hochstadt, N., & Yost, D. (1989). The health care-child welfare partnership: Transitioning medically complex children to the community. *Children's Health Care, 18,* 4-11.

Lynch, M. (1990). Home care of the ventilator-dependent child. *Children's Health Care, 19,* 169-173.

Murray, J. (1989). Payment mechanisms for pediatric home care. *Caring,* October, 33-35.

Quint, R., Chesterman, E., Crain, L., Winkleby, M., & Boyce, T. (1990). Home care for ventilator dependent children. *American Journal of Diseases of Children, 144,* 1238-1241.

Scharer, K., & Dixon, D. (1989). Managing chronic illness: parents with a ventilator-dependent child. *Journal of Pediatric Nursing, 4,* 236-247.

Schreiner, M., Donar, M., & Kettrick, R. (1987). Pediatric home mechanical ventilation. *Pediatric Clinics of North America, 34,* 47-60.

Trachtenberg, S. (1992). Caring and coping: The family of a child with disabilities. In M. Batshaw & Y. Perret, *Children with disabilities: A medical primer* (pp. 563-578). Baltimore: Paul H. Brookes.

Wegener, D., & Aday, L. (1989). Home care for ventilator-assisted children: Predicting family stress. *Pediatric Nursing, 16,* 371-376.

APPENDIX 10-A

Suggested Readings

1. Suggested Readings for Health Care Providers

Aday, L., & Wegener, D. (1988). Home care for ventilator-assisted children: Implications for the children, their families and health policy. *Children's Health Care, 17,* 112-120.

Dalton, R. (1985-86). An evolution of emotional problems faced by ventilator-assisted children. *Psychiatric Forum, 13,* 73-81.

Feinberg, E. (1992). The long aftermath: Ethical dilemmas in resource allocation posed by the care of medically fragile young children. *Zero to Three,* 27-31.

Fingerhood, N. (1986, July-August). Discharging high-risk infants and children to the home. *Coordinator,* 17-22.

Frace, R. (1986). Home ventilation: An alternative to institutionalization. *Focus on Critical Care, 13,* 26-34.

Frates, R., Spaingard, M., Smith, O., & Harrison, G. (1985). Outcome of home mechanical ventilation in children. *The Journal of Pediatrics, 106,* 850-856.

Harris, P. (1988). Sometimes pediatrics home care doesn't work. *American Journal of Nursing,* 851-854.

Hayes, V., & Know, J. (1984). The experience of stress in parents of children hospitalized with long-term disabilities. *Journal of Advanced Nursing, 9,* 333-341.

Koops, B. (1988). Commitment to long-term support: Clinical, economic, and ethical issues. *Bronchopulmonary Dysplasia,* 416-431.

Lynch, M. (1990). Home care of the ventilator-dependent child. *Children's Health Care, 19,* 3, 169-173.

Mallory, G., & Stillwell, P. (1991). The ventilator-dependent child: Issues in diagnosis and management. *Archives of Physical Medicine and Rehabilitation, 72,* 43-55.

Patterson, J. (1990, October). *Caregiving and children.* Paper presented at National Conference on Family Caregiving Across the Lifespan. Cleveland, OH.

Perrin, J. (1992). The nature and extent of chronic illness. *Developmental-Behavioral Pediatrics,* 304-308.

Posch, C., & Edwards, P. (1988). The ventilator-dependent child: Challenge and opportunity. *Rehabilitation Nursing, 13,* 15-18.

Trachtenberg, S. (1992). Caring and coping: The family of a child with disabilities. In M. Batshaw & Y. Perret (Eds.), *Children with disabilities: A medical primer* (pp. 563-578). Baltimore: Paul H. Brookes.

Wong, D. (1991). Transition from hospital to home for children with complex medical care. *Journal of Pediatric Oncology Nursing, 8(1),* 3-9.

2. Suggested Readings for Caregivers

Boba, E. (1990). Faithful care for fragile children. *Caring Magazine, 39,* 12, 26-31.

Caddell, D., & Donaldson, J. (1990). Caring for special children. *Caring Magazine, 9,* 12, 22-25.

Kopf, E. (1986). Caring for a ventilator dependent infant. *Intensive Caring Unlimited,* 3-10.

Thomas, R. (1988). The struggle for control between families and health care providers when a child has complex health care needs. *Zero to Three,* 15-18.

Tompkins, C. (1992). The ventilator dependent child. *Continuing Care,* 28-31.

11

Training Caregivers

Joan Dougherty

INTRODUCTION

A positive home environment is important for all children. For this reason, children receiving technological assistance are encouraged to live outside the hospital as soon as they are medically stable. Yet, all children with tracheostomies require constant supervision and frequent monitoring of their respiratory status. Improper care can result in major setbacks in the child's condition, and can even be life threatening. To avoid potential problems and provide the child with a safe home environment, the family must be trained in all aspects of the child's care. Many children are discharged with some home nursing support, but even children receiving continuous, 24-hour-a-day home nursing must rely on family members for their care when the nurse is sick or absent. Uncovered nursing shifts are not uncommon in home care. It is for the child's safety that training the child and/or the youngster's caregivers is so important.

This chapter describes an approach to training caregivers in the physical care of a child with a tracheostomy in the home. The following topics are addressed:

- Training areas
- Concerns of learners and trainers
- Training of caregivers
- Training procedures for routine aspects of tracheostomy care
- Evaluation of training success

TRAINING AREAS

Before training can begin, it is the responsibility of the primary nurse or team of nurses to review the child's needs and develop a **skills checklist.** This checklist should include all the skills that the learner(s) need to master in order to safely care for the child. For example, when reviewing Frank's case (see Chapter 1 for introductory case history), it is evident that his family will need education in areas of well-baby care, feedings, and developmental intervention, in addition to **tracheostomy** care and management. For this child, it would be essential to include all of these skills in the teaching plan.

Nursing staff have the primary responsibility for training, as they work most closely with the families in doing all of the hospital care, but other disciplines may be assigned responsibility for teaching certain skills. For example, a respiratory therapist might train the family members in performing aerosol treatments, with physical and occupational therapists and speech-language pathologists possibly training the family members in individualized therapy interventions. These other disciplines need to develop their own skill checklist for each of the skills that they are teaching. All of the skills should be combined to form the global teaching plan. The teaching plan should be highly individualized and account for all of an individual child's needs.

Skill Domains

For caregivers, learning all aspects of care can be daunting, but it is necessary to master these skills to properly care for the child in the home. Table 11-1 lists the general areas of physical care to be included in the nursing skills checklist in the order in which they are most often taught. Table 11-2 is a sample teaching plan for Frank.

General knowledge of the anatomy of the respiratory tract and physiology of breathing is important to help the caregiver understand what the tracheostomy is and its purpose in respiration. In the discussion of anatomy, it is essential to include the child's ability or inability to speak with the tracheostomy tube and the need for humidification, as the natural upper airway is bypassed by the tracheostomy tube.

Respiratory assessment is a skill integral to the physical care of a child with a tracheostomy. This assessment includes determining a child's respiratory rate, checking vital signs, listening for breath sounds, checking work of breathing, and reporting changes.

TABLE 11-1. Skills checklist for the physical care of children with tracheostomies in the home.

ORDER OF SKILLS	AREAS OF CARE
1.	General anatomy and physiology of breathing
2.	Respiratory assessment
3.	Percussion and postural drainage
4.	Suctioning
5.	Routine tracheostomy care
6.	Tracheostomy change
7.	Emergency tracheostomy procedures
8.	Aerosol treatments
9.	Oxygen delivery/humidification system/mechanical ventilation
10.	CPR training for children with tracheostomies
11.	Cardiorespiratory monitoring/continuous pulse oximetry

TABLE 11-2. Sample teaching plan for Frank's caregivers.

SKILLS	TEACHER/INSTRUCTOR
1. Well baby care/developmental stimulation therapy	Nursing, PT, OT & SLP
2. Anatomy and physiology of breathing	Nursing
3. Anatomy and physiology of eating	Nursing
4. Oral feeding techniques therapy	Nursing, SLP
5. Gstrostomy tube care	Nursing
6. Gastrostomy tube change	Nursing
7. Gastrostomy tube feedings	Nursing
8. Medication administration (oral/tube)	Nursing
9. Temperature/vital signs	Nursing
10. Respiratory assessment	Nursing
11. Percussion and postural drainage	Nursing
12. Suctioning	Nursing
13. Routine tracheostomy care/string change	Nursing
14. Tracheostomy change	Nursing
15. Aerosol treatments	Respiratory Therapy
16. Oxygen delivery/humidification system	Respiratory Therapy
17. Cardiorespiratory monitoring	Nursing, Home Equipment Co.
18. CPR teaching for tracheostomy patient	Nursing
19. Emergency tracheostomy procedures	Nursing
20. Other:	

Changes are determined by comparing the child's respiratory status at a given time to the child's baseline. Because many children with tracheostomy tubes have concurrent lung disease, their baseline respiratory status may differ from that of a healthy child. For instance, the respiratory rate may be higher than typical for the child's age or the child may adapt by using accessory muscles to assist in breathing. To learn the child's baseline status, the caregiver must spend time evaluating the child's respiratory status while sleeping/awake, at quiet play, and at levels of both moderate and high activity.

All children with tracheostomies require suctioning to keep the tracheostomy tubes patent to maintain a working airway. The child's need for suctioning will vary among children and with circumstance, but the training should focus on average frequency of suctioning and the given child's usual tolerance of the procedure. **Percussion and postural drainage (P & PD)** helps to loosen a child's secretions to allow coughing or suctioning to clear the tracheostomy tube. For children who do not tolerate P & PD, vibration may be an alternate approach to help move a child's secretions.

Aerosol treatments can be given by nebulizer or multidose inhalers. Caregivers must be instructed in the use of the nebulizer or inhaler, as well as the use, indication, and side effects of any medication(s) that it delivers.

Caregivers must be instructed in routine tracheostomy care, including daily care of the child's tracheostomy tube and of the skin at the tracheostomy site on the child's neck. The specifics of procedures depend largely on the type of tracheostomy tube, the type of tracheostomy ties used (Velcro or cloth strings), and the condition of the child's skin around the tracheostomy **stoma** and neck.

Familiarity in performing tracheostomy tube changes and knowledge of emergency procedures is critical for all caregivers of children with tracheostomies. This knowledge includes specialized cardiopulmonary resuscitation (CPR) training. Caregivers with general CPR certification also need specialized training, as the primary airway for resuscitation will likely be the trachea. For some children, such as those with **laryngeal diversions,** a tracheal airway method may be the only way to resuscitate. Common emergencies include accidental **decannulations,** mucous plugs blocking the tracheostomy tube, accidental entry of water into the tracheostomy tube, and difficult tracheostomy insertions that may prolong the time the tracheostomy tube is out of the child. Emergency procedures should be emphasized and should be reviewed frequently—especially just before discharge. The child may be at home for a long time before the caregiver has to deal with an emergency; therefore, all procedures must be routinely reviewed.

Children with tracheostomies typically rely on sophisticated medical equipment, including oxygen delivery systems, humidification systems, **mechanical ventilation,** cardiorespiratory (CR) monitors, and **pulse oximeters.** Depending on the child's medical condition, the youngster will require different levels of respiratory support. For instance, Frank's caregivers needed to learn the tracheostomy humidification system, emergency oxygen use, and a CR monitor for home care. If he had been discharged sooner, his caregivers would have also needed to master the use of additional equipment, including an advanced oxygen delivery system, a pulse oximeter, and a mechanical ventilator. In caring for these children, the learners must be able to operate, monitor, and troubleshoot all equipment as expertly as a respiratory therapist.

LEARNERS AND TRAINERS

Concerns of Caregivers

Jennings (1988) reports that caregivers of children with tracheostomies became concerned when their practical training was not accompanied by written instructions to complement their instruction. It has also been found that many caregivers have a better understanding of the procedures when they are able to read about techniques and/or have illustrations to refer to. Therefore, teaching materials written at about the 6-grade reading level (same as average newspapers) are useful teaching tools. Two sample manuscripts for caregiver teaching booklets on **bronchopulmonary dysplasia (BPD)** are provided in Appendix 11-A and 11-B. Such written summaries would be valuable aids for caregivers of children such as Lisa or Frank to help them understand an underlying disease such as BPD.

Many caregivers in Jennings' (1988) study reported that the training they received helped to meet their own needs, but did not influence relatives, friends, or the child's siblings. Many caregivers interviewed felt isolated as solely responsible in becoming knowledgeable of their child's care. The caregivers felt that videotapes or "real life" photographs could have been used to expose other family members to a child's needs. Such mechanisms may have merit in helping extended families overcome the intimidation about volunteering to help care for children who are technology-assisted.

Another common complaint from caregivers at home is that the home equipment is often very different from the hospital equipment models on which they were taught. Although medical supply companies send a respiratory therapist to the home to review equipment at the child's discharge, the caregivers in the Jennings' (1988) study felt it would have been easier to have been taught on the home equipment from the beginning. Therefore, whenever possible, it is recommended that the home equipment be in the hospital for predischarge caregiver instruction.

Jennings' study (1986) also confirmed the importance of home passes for children approaching discharge. Caregivers of youngsters without home passes before discharge reported traumatic first nights at home. Caregivers whose children had home passes found the trips helpful in smoothing their child's adjustment to home. Lastly, caregivers reported that, despite excellent training, it required about 4 weeks for the child to be at home for caregivers to feel comfortable with providing care. Some reported it took months before they felt confident.

Concerns of Nurses

Nurses, in general, report that caregiver training is a great responsibility, because the nurse is empowering the caregiver to safely care for the child. In many situations, nurses become frustrated when families miss scheduled teaching sessions and fail to see the importance of classes. This is especially possible in a family such as Frank's. In his family's case, the missed teaching sessions may have meant many things: difficulty with transportation, issues at home, ambivalence about actually learning the care, mother using drugs again, or other causes. It is most important for the social worker to work with the nurse(s) in dealing with these issues early (see Chapter 10). Even the best teaching plan cannot succeed without cooperation and commitment from the family.

In Frank's case, a **teaching contract** with the family could have been developed (see Appendix 11-C for a sample teaching contract). In the contract, the caregivers would negotiate the plan with the teaching nurses. The contract would include the teaching plan, the schedule for teaching days, identified persons to learn care and a time frame for the teaching. Other items to include in a training plan for Frank might be transportation arrangements and how the family was to handle missed teaching sessions. These contracts are reviewed and signed by the learners. The contracts are not legally binding, but they assist the learning process.

TRAINING PROCEDURES

Identification of Learners and Trainers

Health care providers most typically train caregivers of infants, along with family members or friends of the family to care for the children at home. Some older children with tracheostomies are able to assist their caretakers and may become independent in much of their care (see Chapter 12). It is recommended that a minimum of two people learn all the care to assist each other at home and give one another a break when they are tired, ill, or otherwise incapacitated.

Ideally, all family members should learn basic medical procedures to ensure the child's safety and, most importantly, to encourage family socialization, along with participation in the child's care. In families with one caregiver, such as Frank's, one often finds that family members, such a grandparents, are willing to be additional caregivers. Because of the complexity of the child's care, children with single caregivers who have no back-up support are not usually discharged to home. Discharging a child with only one caregiver, even with increased home nursing support, most often has discouraging results. In a few cases, the end result will be rehospitalization of the child because of caregiver stress and inability to cope.

In most busy hospital units, several nurses conduct the predischarge training. Therefore, the teaching plan and the student needs should be in writing for all the trainers to refer to. Caregivers can become confused when each nurse presents a different method of performing a skill. For example, there are many ways to tie tracheostomy strings, therefore, the nurse developing the teaching plan should select the best way for that particular child and family and communicate the scheduled method in writing to the other nurses. This assures consistency in the teaching and alleviates student frustration and confusion.

Initial Training

Once the students have been identified, with the skills checklist and teaching plan individualized to the child's home care needs, the training can officially begin. At this point, depending on the time it took to identify students' needs, the home caregivers may have already begun learning some aspects of the care through observation and handling of the child. It is important at this time to review with the students all of the skills that will be included in the training and order that the skills will be presented. A general guideline for the order of skills necessary to care for a child with a tracheostomy is found in the skills checklist (Table 11-1). In some instances, a caregiver may have already started to learn the use of the CR monitor, but is still frightened of working with the tracheostomy tube. In this case, it is better to review the CR monitor early in the teaching plan to help build confidence and allow students to become comfortable with providing the care.

It is equally important to discuss with each student the method by which they best learn. This helps the nurse to identify the learning style of the individual and consider what teaching methods will work best. Some persons will indicate a few preferred methods rather than one method. This should be encouraged, because the nurse has many different skills to teach—some being concrete (e.g., tracheostomy care), and some being abstract (e.g., anatomy and physiology of breathing). Employing methods that mesh with the individual's learning style is the best way to achieve success. Questions that can assist the nurse in identifying the preferred learning style include: Does the student read well? Does the person find video tapes helpful? Would the caregiver prefer to work with dolls at first? Does the student like to review procedures in writing before observing them?

Fortunately, although medical procedures for children with tracheostomies are complex, most adults are capable of learning the care procedures if the learning material is presented in a sequence of small logical steps, tailored to the learner's needs (Kennelly, 1990). Although having good manual dexterity helps, determination and commitment are the principal requirements for learning the necessary medical procedures. It is difficult to predict the training time required, as needs and aptitude differ greatly from family to family. Some families learn all the training in as little as 2 weeks, but that is the exception, not the norm. However, it is certain that an organized teaching plan shortens the time it takes to train the family for home care.

Teaching Sessions

Caregivers may schedule their teaching sessions individually or together. Teaching certain skills may require individual instruction; but learning with others, especially the support people, has positive aspects. Teaching the caregivers together helps foster cooperation in the child's home care, may increase their motivation to learn, and builds confidence in one another's abilities. Teaching tracheostomy tube changes or tracheostomy emergency procedures to the group helps them prepare for the future when they will need to work as a team to successfully complete these procedures. However, there are times when group learning may not be beneficial. For example, if one student has difficulty remembering steps to a procedure and performs out of sequence repeatedly, it may influence another student, who might start to confuse the steps, as well. In such a case, individual instruction may get both learners on the "right track" until they are ready to try the procedure together. Personalized instruction allows the nurse to focus on the individual's learning style and needs. It allows flexibility, individualized pacing of the sessions, and makes the student a "real" part of the process (de Tornyay & Thompson, 1987). It helps students succeed on their own and builds confidence, as well.

Teaching Tools

It is best to develop a list of teaching tools as part of the teaching plan. This should be based on learning style and preferred teaching methods, as well as individual versus group learning needs. For instance, teaching concepts such as anatomy and physiology of breathing will require some visualization of the respiratory tract, along with verbal explanations. The use of drawings or models can be very helpful. Teaching well-baby care may not require any teaching tools other than "hands on" practice with the child in the presence of the nurse. When teaching a highly technical skill, such as suctioning or tracheostomy change, it is best to begin with simulation on a doll and progress to "hands on" with the child once the student is comfortable with the procedure. Some skills will require total simulation, such as CPR. Using the CPR mannequin with a tracheostomy tube in place has proven most helpful.

Teaching tools include caregiver teaching booklets, videotapes, audiotapes, models, drawings, and practice dolls. Sometimes it is necessary to use some or all of these tools in combination. Most caregivers learning tracheostomy home care prefer to have the procedure demonstrated several times before they feel ready to try it themselves. With tracheostomy changes and tracheostomy string changes, success has been achieved using videotapes of these procedures and dolls with tracheostomies for "pretraining" sessions. This allows the caregivers to observe and practice without worrying that they may accidentally hurt the child. Audiotapes of breath sounds have helped students identify abnormal breath sounds, such as **wheezing** or **rales.** They will need to identify these sounds if their child becomes sick, but may not be able to hear them when listening to their well child in the hospital.

Simulation of procedures or situations is a necessary teaching method. Simulation allows the real situation to be experienced without risk to the child, and the experiences can be repeated as often as desired or can be interrupted for discussion. It is important to set up the role plays as close to the real life situation as possible. Using tools (dolls, models, equipment, etc.) enhances any simulation. For instance, one might set up simulation for tracheostomy emergency procedures by using a doll with the same type of tracheostomy and emergency equipment the child will have at home. The student should be encouraged to respond to the simulation as if the doll is the "real" child and the alarms are also "real." The nurse then sets up varying scenarios, allowing the simulation experience to cover potential problems or difficulties that might arise when working with a "real" child. The nurse should provide the students with feedback on the likely consequences of their actions. The sequence of activities should be sufficient to assure that the procedures practiced will transfer to "real" situations (de Tornyay & Thompson, 1987).

Hands-on training should begin when the student feels ready. Some caregivers prefer to begin the teaching plan with hands-on training, with others taking weeks of stimulation practice before they are ready. In hands-on training, it is essential that the nurse work closely with the student and child to assure safety and assist as needed. It is recommended that a caregiver observe the nurse doing the procedure at least once with the child before attempting to assist the nurse. Of course, there are procedures (such as CPR and emergency procedures) that will never be practiced with the child unless an emergency situation arises during the training session.

PROCEDURES FOR TRAINING CAREGIVERS IN ROUTINE ASPECTS OF TRACHEOSTOMY CARE

Whether using simulation or hands-on training, the students should observe the procedure(s), demonstrate the procedure(s), and review the procedure(s) until they have achieved the expected outcome—for example, three successful tracheostomy tube changes. In teaching the skills, nurses should demonstrate procedures step-by-step, keeping the information as basic as possible to avoid overwhelming the caregiver. Breaking the procedures into three phases can assist the student. In a preparation phase the student is encouraged to gather all necessary equipment before starting a procedure—helping them to be organized and minimizing the amount of time that the procedure will take with a child, who may get upset or restless. The procedure phase includes breaking each step of the procedure into small basic steps. Procedural explanations can be as basic or as detailed as the caregiver needs. The concluding behavior phase includes any necessary follow-up steps, for instance, reapplying the child's CR monitor after a bath or reporting changes to the physician after a respiratory assessment. This phase also includes proper disposal of old materials and returning of supplies and equipment to proper places for easy access later. If the student observes the procedures in this fashion, it makes it easier for them to understand, practice, and eventually demonstrate the procedures before the habituation in home care.

Table 11-1 lists the needed training areas. Detailed description of procedures for all areas is beyond the scope of a single chapter. The next sections include procedures for more routine aspects of tracheostomy care, including P&PD and suctioning for a child who is both tracheostomized and ventilator-assisted, and routine tracheostomy care (care of the tracheostomy site and string change) for a child with a tracheostomy who may or may not also receive ventilator assistance. Chapter 12 describes procedures to train older children to self-suction.

Percussion and Postural Drainage

Preparation

1. Perform respiratory assessment.
2. Note if child needs P&PD to loosen and move secretions from the lower lungs by listening with stethoscope during respiratory assessment procedure.
3. Avoid feeding child for 1 hour before P&PD.
4. Obtain laerdal bag attached to oxygen.
5. Turn oxygen on.
6. Check that oxygen is on and flowing through laerdal bag.
7. Obtain a towel or light blanket.
8. Completely wash surface of hands with soap and water, with no dirt or residue visible and thoroughly dry.

Procedure

1. Disconnect child's ventilator tubing from tracheostomy connector.
2. Cork ventilator tubing.
3. Attach laerdal bag to child's tracheostomy connector.
4. Squeeze laerdal bag and release four times.
5. Disconnect laerdal bag and place nearby.
6. Remove cork from ventilation tubing.
7. Attach ventilation tubing to tracheostomy connector.
8. Position child **supine,** with head lower than trunk in bed or in lap.
9. Place towel or blanket over chest area to be percussed.
10. Cup hands.
11. Clap hands in cupped position between collarbone and

nipple on each side of chest, for approximately 3 minutes on each side.
12. Check that clapping is vigorous, but not painful.
13. Check that a slapping sound is not heard. If a slap is heard, cup hands more and continue.
14. Turn child on one side with head downward.
15. Clap hands in cupped position over the ribs just below the armpit for approximately 3 minutes.
16. Turn child to other side with head downward.
17. Clap hands in cupped position over the ribs just below the armpit on this side.
18. Turn child on stomach with head down.
19. Clap hands in cupped position over middle of back below shoulder blade and on both sides of spine for approximately 3 minutes each side.
20. Be sure not to clap over spine, chest, bone, or below ribs.
21. Sit child upright.

Concluding Behaviors

1. Proceed with suctioning.
2. Perform respiratory assessment.

Suctioning

Preparation

1. Check for any signs that suctioning is required, including: noisy breathing, coughing or gurgling of secretions, and pale or bluish lips, nail beds, or skin color.
2. Always follow P&PD with suction.
3. Place suction machine in reach of the person treating the child for the procedure.
4. Test that suction machine works when turned on.
5. Turn suction machine off.
6. Obtain suction catheter of correct size for child's tracheostomy.
7. Open suction catheter package.
8. Connect plastic end of catheter to suction machine tubing, leaving the catheter itself inside the package.
9. Obtain a clean paper cup and rubber gloves.
10. Obtain a sterile water bottle and remove lid.
11. Pour 1-2 oz. of sterile water into the paper cup.
12. Replace lid on sterile water bottle.
13. Obtain a saline vial.

14. Open saline vial.
15. Place laerdal bag attached to oxygen in reach of the child.
16. Turn on oxygen.
17. Check that oxygen is on and flowing through the bag.
18. Completely wash surface of hands with soap and water until no dirt or residue is visible, then dry.

Procedure

1. Disconnect ventilator tubing from child's tracheostomy connector.
2. Attach laerdal bag to child's tracheostomy connector.
3. Put cork in ventilator tubing.
4. Press alarm reset.
5. Squeeze laerdal bag with hand and release.
6. Squeeze and release laerdal bag two more times. If child is breathless or color is pale or blue, squeeze and release bag until child returns to normal color.
7. Put on gloves.
8. Squeeze and release laerdal bag again.
9. Remove the screw cap from the child's tracheostomy.
10. Put 2-3 drops of saline into the screw-cap opening of the tracheostomy.
11. Cover the opening with your finger.
12. Keeping your finger in place, use your other hand to squeeze laerdal bag.
13. Let go of bag.
14. Move your finger off screw-cap opening.
15. Turn on suction.
16. Remove suction catheter from package without touching the end of the catheter on the child, bedding, or other materials.
17. Insert catheter into the screw-cap opening just 1 mm past the length of the tracheostomy tube.
18. Put thumb of other hand over suction catheter hole to begin suction.
19. Slowly rotate catheter while pulling it out of the opening in 10 seconds or less while applying intermittent pressure over suction hole with your thumb.
20. Hold your own breath while pulling suction catheter out to help you feel the need to remove it.
21. Coil suction catheter around hand that you just used to insert catheter into opening; do not allow the end to touch anything but your glove.

22. Immediately cover the screw-cap opening with a finger of your hand that has the coiled suction catheter in it.
23. Using your other hand, squeeze and release the laerdal bag 4 times.
24. Remove your finger from screw-cap opening. Uncoil suction catheter from that hand, keeping the end of the catheter in the same hand.
25. Place the end of suction catheter that you just suctioned with in cup of sterile water.
26. Put thumb of other hand over suction catheter hole to begin suction.
27. Continue to suction up water until catheter is clear of secretions.
28. Immediately cover the screw-cap opening with a finger of your hand, holding the end of the suction catheter.
29. Using your other hand, squeeze and release laerdal bag 2 times.
30. Insert suction catheter again as previously instructed and repeat steps 17-27, until you can suction no more secretions from tracheostomy.
31. After cleaning catheter with sterile water in step 27 following final suction, hold catheter in hand and turn glove inside out over catheter.
32. Screw cap back over opening on tracheostomy.
33. Squeeze and release laerdal bag 2 times.
34. Remove laerdal bag.
35. Remove cork from ventilator tubing. Place cork in container near ventilator.
36. Attach ventilator tubing to child's tracheostomy connector.
37. Follow up with respiratory assessment procedures.

Concluding Behaviors

1. Discard gloves and catheter into trash receptacle.
2. Insert suction machine tubing into cup of water to rinse tubing.
3. Return suction machine tubing to suction machine. Turn off suction machine.
4. Discard paper cup in trash receptacle.
5. Discard saline vial in tracheostomy receptacle.
6. Return laerdal bag to proper place.
7. Turn oxygen off.
8. Rinse out suction canister with soap and water and dry.
9. Return suction machine to proper place.

Care of the Tracheostomy

Preparation

1. Place trash receptacle nearby.
2. Pour clean water into a paper cup.
3. Obtain Q-tips.
4. Obtain 3 clean gauze pads (4 × 4″).
5. Remove child's shirt to expose neck area.
6. Completely wash surface of hands with soap and water, with no dirt or residue visible, then dry.

Procedure

1. Remove old gauze pads from under child's tracheostomy phalanges.
2. Inspect neck area for any signs of redness, irritation, or drainage.
3. Dip Q-tip in cup of water.
4. Wipe area around one side of the tracheostomy stoma, moving the Q-tip from the stoma towards the neck.
5. Discard this Q-tip in trash receptacle.
6. Dip clean Q-tip in water cup.
7. Wipe area around the other side of the stoma, moving the Q-tip from the stoma towards the neck.
8. Discard this Q-tip in trash receptacle.
9. Dry areas on both sides of stoma with clean gauze pad.
10. Fold 4 × 4″ gauze pad in half.
11. Place this pad under the phalange, keeping the folded side toward the stoma.
12. Fold another 4 × 4″ gauze pad in half.
13. Place this pad under the other phalange, keeping the folded side toward the stoma.
14. Straighten both pads so that an even/equal amount of each pad is above and below the phalange.

Concluding Behaviors

1. Put child's shirt back on.
2. Discard old gauze pads and water cup in trash receptacle.
3. Completely wash surface of hands with soap and water, with no dirt or residue visible, then dry.
4. Report any increased irritation or drainage to the child's doctor.

String Change

Preparation

1. Check child's tracheostomy strings for soiling.
2. Flex child's head forward.
3. Place fingers under foam at the back of the child's neck to make certain you can only get 1 finger under foam or padding.
4. Obtain a roll of tracheostomy string or Velcro strings, if the child uses Velcro.
5. Obtain a pair of scissors and hemostats.
6. Obtain a premeasured length of reston foam if the child has regular tracheostomy strings.
7. Obtain two gauze pads (4 × 4″).
8. Remove child's shirt to expose neck area.
9. Completely wash surface of hands with soap and water, with no dirt or residue visible, then dry.

Procedure

1. For regular tracheostomy strings, follow this step 1.a-n. For Velcro, go to step 2. Cut two pieces of tracheostomy string about 10 inches long.
   a. Tie a knot at the end of each string.
   b. Use hemostat or scissors to cut a small, approximately 1 cm slit in each string directly in front of each knot.
   c. Remove old gauze pads.
   d. With old strings in place, place end of new string without the knot through the hole in one side of the tracheostomy phalange.
   e. Pull string through until you reach the slit.
   f. Thread the end through the slit in the string and pull tightly.
   g. Place the other string through the hole of the other side of the tracheostomy phalange.
   h. Again, pull string through until you reach the slit.
   i. Thread the end through the slit in the string and pull tightly.
   j. Remove paper backing from foam.
   k. Place the middle of one string against the sticky part of the foam.
   l. Fold foam over string so that foams sticks to itself.
   m. Pull the string with the foam attached all the way around the child's neck to the other side.

   n. Tie the two strings on this side in a bow so that the foam rests against the child's neck. Go to step 3.
2. Obtain Velcro string of correct size.
   a. Remove old gauze pads.
   b. With old strings in place, place end of string through the hole in one side of the tracheostomy phalange.
   c. Pull string through until you reach the padding.
   d. Place the other string through the hole of the other side of the tracheostomy phalange.
   e. Again, pull string until you reach the padding.
   f. Pull strings snugly around neck and attach Velcro at end of string to padding. Go to step 3.
3. Flex child's head forward.
4. Place fingers under new foam at the back of the child's neck to make certain you can only get 1 finger under foam.
5. If more than one finger fits under foam or padding, untie and tighten. Retie and check again.
6. If it is too tight to fit one finger under foam or padding, untie and loosen strings. Retie and check again.
7. If only one finger fits under foam or padding, pull both loops of bow till they form a knot for regular strings or leave Velcro strings fastened as is.
   a. For regular strings, tie strings in two more knots and cut extra strings on each side of knot leaving only 2-3 inches.
   b. For Velcro, leave fastened as is.
8. Cut old strings being careful not to sever new strings or tracheostomy phalanges.
9. Remove all pieces of old string from phalange.
10. If new strings are cut, remove the new strings from the phalanges, and repeat the procedure.
11. If phalange is cut, the tracheostomy tube must be changed immediately.
12. Fold a 4 × 4″ gauze pad in half.
13. Place folded side of gauze pad against tracheostomy stoma while inserting pad under one side of the phalange.
14. Fold the other 4 × 4″ gauze pad in half.
15. Place this pad under the other phalange while keeping the folded side toward the stoma.

Concluding Behaviors

1. Put child's shirt back on.
2. Discard old gauze pads and strings in trash receptacle.
3. Return scissors, hemostats, tracheostomy strings, and foam to proper places.

TRAINING EVALUATION

Before a caregiver is considered to be trained and prepared for home care, return demonstrations must be performed with the nurse present until the student has mastered a skill to the nurses' satisfaction. It is recommended that a caregiver demonstrate each skill correctly at least three times to demonstrate "skill mastery." In general, repeating a skill three times is usually sufficient practice, but some caregivers may not feel comfortable with certain skills, such as a tracheostomy tube change, until their fifth or sixth time.

Although the student's demonstration of mastery of skills is required, the nurse, as the evaluator, should further evaluate the caregiver's ability to generalize skills to new situations that might arise at home. For instance, a student may be able to explain a child's need for tracheostomy tube humidification based on the caregiver's knowledge of the anatomy of the respiratory tract. If the humidifier is broken, however, does the caregiver know how long the child could go without humidity, or what steps to take while waiting for a new humidification system? It is the teacher's responsibility to challenge the caregiver to extend knowledge for such situations that may happen at home.

The final trial for evaluation is to simulate the home experience while still in the hospital, such as having child and caregiver in an independent living apartment, or by providing short passes for the child to receive home care. This, of course, requires that training be completed, because the caregivers will be independently responsible for all of the care. In a hospital apartment situation, caregivers can be responsible for all of the child's care, with the hospital staff nearby. Home passes can be a step closer to home and should be encouraged whenever possible. If these situations are not successful, retraining will be necessary. Often, caregivers will be able to identify previously unknown areas that need review, after a pass or apartment stay.

CONCLUSIONS

Children's hospitals are confronting the challenge of caring for a growing number of children with tracheostomy tubes. Many less specialized hospitals face the same challenge. Recognizing that hospitals are often not the best settings for the physical and psychosocial development of these children, hospitals have implemented discharge teaching programs for the families of these children. To a great extent, the quality of home care is dependent on the success of the teaching program and the level of comfort the family has with the child's care.

The training required for a caregiver to manage the physical home care of a child who has been tracheostomized is extensive and requires commitment by the student(s). Having an organized teaching plan is a key component in the learning process. The teaching plan described in this chapter has been used successfully to teach many different caregivers, including those with reading difficulties, poor educations, and mild learning disabilities.

REFERENCES

de Tornyay, R., & Thompson, M.A, (1987). *Strategies for teaching nursing* (3rd ed.). New York: John Wiley & Sons.

Jennings, P. (1988). Nursing and home aspects of the care of a child with a tracheostomy. *Journal of Laryngology and Otology,* (Suppl. 17), 25-29.

Kennelly, C. (1990). Tracheostomy care: Parents as learners. *The Journal of Maternal/Child Nursing,* 2, 264-267.

APPENDIX 11-A

Bronchopulmonary Dysplasia Caregiver Teaching Booklet

BPD is a respiratory condition that can occur in very premature infants or infants who have been treated for distress with high amounts of oxygen and/or high pressure ventilation for long periods. Usually the child's airway and lungs (the respiratory system) improve with time as they grow. Following recovery, the child may catch respiratory infections more easily and may have limited energy for exercise. Children with BPD require special care. Families can learn to care for their children at home with help from their physician.

SIGNS AND SYMPTOMS

Some things your doctor may look for:

• Abnormal chest X-ray
• Increased breathing rate and effort
• Need for oxygen (may need mechanical ventilation)
• High amounts of carbon dioxide (CO_2) in the blood.

SPECIAL CARE

1. OXYGEN THERAPY

If the child is unable to get enough oxygen on his/her own, the oxygen in the blood decreases and the child must breathe harder and faster. Giving oxygen therapy allows the child to rest and breathe comfortably. Oxygen is like a drug and must be given in the amount your doctor orders. A more detailed book will be provided.

2. FLUID MANAGEMENT

Many children with BPD have trouble controlling their fluid output. They require drugs or limiting fluids to prevent excess fluids. Things to look for:

• Less urine in diapers or urinating less than usual
• Puffiness, especially around hands, feet, or eyes
• Extra amounts of fluids taken in
• Medication doses missed

Excess fluid usually leads to difficult breathing and increased heart and respiratory rates. "Rales," or crackling sounds, may be heard when listening to the lungs with a stethoscope. (To imagine rales, rub pieces of hair together by your ear.) Your doctor should be called if you notice these signs. Treatment is necessary.

Diuretics are medications used to prevent excess fluids. Common medications include Lasix, Diuril and Aldactone. These are prescriptions by your doctor and must be given as ordered. Some diuretics affect the body's level of potassium, which is needed for good health. Therefore, KCL or another potassium medication will also be ordered. It is important that your child gets these medications even though they taste bad.

3. NUTRITION

Children with BPD use much of their energy to breathe and they tire easily during feedings. It is important to watch your child's growth and follow your doctor's suggestions. Often these children need a high-calorie formula or are given high-calorie additives in their bottles. Some children will require tube feedings to increase their calories. If there is no other medical problem, the tube feedings should only be temporary. Our staff can provide tube feeding instruction.

4. DEVELOPMENT

Many BPD children were very ill at birth and some delays in their growth and development are expected. It is very important to remember that many of these children are restricted from regular activities because they tire easily or are limited because they need oxygen. You should encourage activities without overtiring your child. Your child will probably receive some therapy at home. Physical and occupational therapists can provide suggestions for you to use with your child.

5. RESPIRATORY ASSESSMENT

A detailed book will be provided.

APPENDIX 11-B

Respiratory Assessment Booklet

When assessing your child's respiratory status, it is very important to know your youngster's "usual" status. Many areas need to be checked. It is important that an assessment is done frequently throughout the day.

DEFINITIONS

RESPIRATORY RATE	Number of breaths per minute. May be counted by watching belly move or by listening with a stethoscope.
RETRACTIONS	Appearance of skin being pulled between ribs and/or above and below breastbone.
NASAL FLARING	Flaring of outer sides of nose with inspiration.
WHEEZE	"Squeak" heard on either inspiration or expiration. Usually heard if the child's airway has narrowed.

YOU SHOULD KNOW

1. Child's usual respiratory rate both awake and asleep.
2. If the child has retraction or shows signs of increased breathing effort with activity,
3. How the child's breathing sounds with a stethoscope.

PROCEDURE

With a stethoscope, listen to your child's lungs while breathing normally. Listen for at least one full breath in each location. Breath sounds should be listened to in the front and the back of the child's chest. Avoid areas such as the shoulder blades and breastbone. While listening, compare side to side. Breath sounds will be louder near the top of the chest and decrease as you go lower. By hospital discharge, you should be comfortable in your familiarity with your child's breath sounds.

THINGS TO LOOK FOR

1. Increased respiratory rate
2. Increased retractions
3. Nasal flaring
4. Blue color of nailbeds and/or lips
5. Pale or blue skin color
6. Decreased breath sounds in the lungs
7. Wheezing or crackling sounds heard with a stethoscope

With any signs of distress, try to determine the cause. Sometimes rest or proper oxygen (if used) is the solution. Other times your child may require extra respiratory treatments. These include percussion, medications, and other procedures that the nursing team will teach you as needed for your child.

APPENDIX 11-C

Sample Teaching Contract

In preparing to safely care for your child at home, you will need special training to learn and demonstrate the required care. This is a special and sometimes difficult task. It will require many teaching and practice sessions. The amount of time it will take for you to learn these skills varies. In order to complete the training as soon as possible so that your child can go home, you must meet the following conditions:

1. Primary student and/or back-up student needs to be present for each teaching session.
2. Teaching sessions will occur (*day*) and (*day*) at (*time*) each week and primary learner must be at 6 out of 8 teaching sessions in a 1-month period.
3. If unable to attend a session, you must call (*telephone number*) before 9 a.m.
4. If transportation is a problem, Social Work staff will assist you.
5. No siblings may be present for the teaching session. Social Work will assist you in arranging childcare, when possible.
6. Students must correctly perform each skill according to our teaching protocol.

Things to learn:

1. Well-child care.
2. Vital signs (temperature, pulse, respirations).
3. Respiratory
   a. Assessment
   b. Treatments
   c. P & PD
   d. Suction
4. Tracheostomy care
   a. Site care

   b. String change
   c. Tracheostomy change & emergency care
5. CR monitor
6. CPR
7. Developmental intervention
   a. Therapies
   b. Hearing aid
   c. Suggested play activities

Facts to consider:

1. The equipment may be noisy. At home, you may wish to put your child in a separate bedroom, with monitoring at all times.
2. Your electric bill may double. Amounts depend on your home, type of machinery, and hours of use per day.
3. You will need to spend your own money on supplies, such as paper cups, diapers, formula, sterilizing water.
4. You will lose some of your privacy. Nurses and therapists will be visiting your home on a scheduled basis.

I understand that the foregoing information is necessary for me to learn in order to safely care for my child at home. I identify the back-up person to be _____ . We agree to complete the teaching with the staff as outlined in this teaching contract. I understand that my participation and progress in learning the care will be documented and the results shared with me.

_____   _____
Caregiver(s) signature   Social Worker's signature

_____   _____
Back-Up signature   Nursing Care Coordinator signature

                                              _____
                                              Attending M.D. signature

                                              _____
                                              Witness

12

Training Children

John M. Parrish

INTRODUCTION

Throughout this book, considerable importance has been assigned to what a well-coordinated team of professionals can offer to children who are technologically assisted. The importance of the roles and responsibilities of various professionals in the lives of these children can not be denied. Nonetheless, dependence for care by the patient often prompts the notion that professionals, more so than the child and family, are entrusted to take actions necessary to protect the child's well-being, with the child and family passively participating in recommended chronic care protocols.

However, as societal trends contribute to a heightened concern for the civil rights of citizens with developmental disabilities, and there is more widespread acceptance of the significance of technological advances and the patient's overall ecology, there is increasing recognition that individuals who are assisted by technology also want to be included in and empowered by the selection and conduct of their care regimens. Correspondingly, secondary to promoting the ongoing survival and development of the child with a tracheostomy, the principal goal of habilitation is to enable the child and family to self-administer prescribed medical regimens with proficiency in least restrictive, community-referenced settings (e.g., homes and schools), without excessive reliance on or interference by professional care providers. When this child- and family-centered goal is achieved, or at least approximated, the child and family are better able to participate in the mainstream of society and to enjoy more independent lives with fewer social and economic encumbrances.

Toward that purpose, this section concludes with a discussion of how a child might be taught to manage aspects of daily self care. The children who are appropriate candidates for this training typically are 4 years or older in cognitive development, do not have physical disabilities that would make self-care impossible, and are emotionally "ready" to assume more responsibility for their care as judged by the child, caregivers, and professional staff. Self-suctioning is used to illustrate how training a child to manage aspects of daily care might be achieved. However, the competency-based approach described in this chapter might also be used to train appropriate children, caregivers, and paraprofessionals to perform all of the daily care activities described in Chapter 11.

The following topics are addressed in this chapter:

- Importance of developing self-care skills
- Competency based training
- Designing and conducting a competency-based curriculum
- Motivational systems
- Evaluating outcomes of competency-based curricula
- Efficiency of competency-based training
- Social validation of competency-based curricula

IMPORTANCE OF DEVELOPING SELF-CARE SKILLS

Children with special health needs, including those with tracheostomies, require skilled care on a daily basis (Stool & Beebe, 1973). The under-skilled child with a tracheostomy often depends on adult care providers who are trained professionals to accomplish prescribed routines in a competent, timely manner (Kennedy, Johnson, & Sturdevant, 1982). In the absence of this skilled adult care, the child's vulnerability to disease or disability increases significantly (Schreiner, Donar, & Kettrick, 1987; Singer, Wood, & Lambert, 1985). However, provision of skilled care by professionals not only involves maintenance of necessary routines to sustain children's health and to promote the child's further growth and development, it also entails teaching children to become progressively competent in the conduct of the routines themselves (Derrickson, Neef, & Parrish, 1991).

Skill acquisition by patients ultimately lessens the burden and cost of child care (Riley, Parrish, & Cataldo, 1989). For example, as children who are technologically assisted and their families become more skilled in the completion of **tracheostomy** care, less time and effort is required for the satisfactory conduct of care routines (Bosch & Cuyler, 1987; Jennings, 1988; Ruben et al., 1982). Collaterally, there is less need for incessant, expensive care by paid professionals (Friedman, 1986).

Skill mastery may also contribute to the child's and family's sense of self-efficacy, in that those with skills may exercise greater control over what happens to them and may be better able to enjoy more independent and private lives (Singer & Irvin, 1989). Achievement of competency in regard to self-directed tracheostomy care may also enhance the likelihood that the child will be able to participate in other skill training programs available in environments less restrictive than hospitals, nursing homes, or hospices. As is true for other children who are technologically assisted, achievement of functional independence in regard to self-care may enable those youngsters with tracheostomies to participate more fully in the mainstream, such as regular public education (*Tatro* v. *State of Texas*, 1984).

COMPETENCY-BASED TRAINING

The most prevalent method of adult instruction by far has been inservice, or "on-the-job," training provided through workshops (i.e., lectures), directed readings, focused discussions, and limited supervised practice. Such training may result in transient improvements in the skills of the adult caretakers and indirectly the skills of the children they serve (e.g., Gage, Fredericks, Johnson-Dorn, & Lindley-Southard, 1982; Watson & Uzzell, 1980; Zlomke & Benjamin, 1983). These didactic methods may serve to enhance a student's understanding or "awareness," yet alone are not likely to affect the student's capability to master a specific task by taking a specific action, even when such tasks have been featured during the training (Parrish, Egel, & Neef, 1986; Ziarnik & Bernstein, 1982). Furthermore, when these didactic practices are extended to children, the methods are even less effective than they are with adults.

One promising alternative, or supplement, to the aforementioned training methods is a **competency-based training paradigm** (Calkins, Gibson, Grosko, & Bueker, 1982; Lukenbill et al., 1976). Within such a paradigm, greatest emphasis is placed on the acquisition and maintenance of specific skills by the student, in contrast to a focus on the sharing of general information designed to improve the student's attitudes or knowledge base. The key philosophical underpinning of this approach is that "one learns best by doing." Training focuses on "how to do what when." This approach applies as equally well to children as to adults.

Through well-controlled clinical trials, competency-based training curricula have been demonstrated repeatedly to be efficacious as a means of training caregivers to care for their children with handicaps (e.g., Feldman, Manella, & Varni, 1983; Gross, Eudy, & Drabman, 1982; Jenkins, Stephens, Sternberg, 1980; Macy, Solomon, Schoen, & Galey, 1983; O'Dell, Blackwell, Larcen, & Hogan, 1977; Rickert et al., 1988; Salzinger, Feldman, & Portnoy, 1970; Sandler, Coren, & Thurman, 1983; Weitz, 1981). With increasing frequency, a competency-based methodology is being employed to teach young children with developmental disabilities how to self-administer prescribed medical regimens (e.g., Babbitt, Parrish, Brierley, & Kohr, 1991; Derrickson, Neef, & Parrish, 1991; Neef, Parrish, Hannigan, Page, & Iwata, 1986; Richman, Ponticas, Page, & Epps, 1986).

DESIGNING AND CONDUCTING A COMPETENCY-BASED CURRICULUM

The defining characteristics of a competency-based curriculum are indicated in Table 12-1.

Identification and Social Validation of Target Skills

In most cases, at the onset of curriculum development and before actual provision of training, the curriculum designer

TABLE 12-1. Defining characteristics of a competency-based curriculum.

STEPS	CHARACTERISTICS OF A COMPETENCY-BASED CURRICULUM
1.	Development of task analyses, corresponding operational definitions, and assessment instruments
2.	Collection of baseline data before training
3.	Specification of student objectives
4.	Provision of systematic training
5.	Completion of skill rehearsals
6.	Repeated measurement of student performance in simulated and criterion (actual) situations
7.	Provision of remedial training, as indicated

pinpoints target skills that must be acquired by participating children and caregivers to meet each child's special health needs. Requisite skills are ascertained typically through consultation with health care providers who routinely deliver services to the particular patient or patients who is/are to participate in training. If, for instance, the training objective is tracheostomy care, the child's attending physician and clinical nurse specialist, in addition to experienced home care nurses, are often the best sources of this consultation.

In addition, the curriculum designer examines the extant literature describing the effective implementation of the relevant management routines by skilled professionals to further refine curricular content. Most importantly, the trainer directly observes professionals, caregivers, and children who have already mastered the target skills. Such ethnological observations reveal the content and sequence of competent performance by those more experienced with the recommended care routines.

Development of Task Analyses, Corresponding Operational Definitions, and Assessment Instruments

A **task analysis** is a step-by-step description of exactly what the child is and is not to do during the prescribed management routine. Each step is behaviorally defined in terms of what the child is to say or do. Each step is an action or set of actions that is observable and measurable. The provisional task analyses derived from the aforementioned procedure are then submitted to a panel of professional experts, experienced caregivers and, on occasion, skilled patients, with a request that they independently judge the relevance and importance of each identified component of the planned curriculum for the quality of care. Revisions to the initial task analysis are then completed, based on the opinions and recommendations of these judges. This process is a critical aspect of assessing the social as well as the content validity of the planned curriculum.

Once the final task analysis is established, an operational definition is developed for each step of the procedure. A companion checklist of the requisite steps to be completed to accomplish the care routine is then created, allowing the trainer to readily assess and quickly indicate if each step is completed correctly in proper sequence by the child during structured skill rehearsals. The procedures presented in Chapter 11 represent a series of steps that might then be made into a companion checklist.

Collection of Baseline Data Before Training

One of the characteristics of competency-based training is that the student's skills are assessed before training commences. The competency-based trainer immediately presents the student with an actual problem-solving vignette designed to require each of the requisite skills for satisfactory resolution of the problem (e.g., a role play of satisfactory completion of a tracheostomy care routine). The assessment is a short series of direct observations of the student's performance of those skills targeted for training. Typically, the trainer gives the child at least three opportunities to demonstrate skill proficiency, using the assessment instrument from the task analysis to score the child's performance.

Often termed **baseline,** this assessment indicates if systematic training is required and, if so, where training efforts could be most profitably directed. Frequently, children demonstrate partial mastery of a task before systematic training, suggesting selected facets of the planned curriculum that can be merely reviewed or skipped altogether, allowing more time for training of the specific skill deficits detected. Hence, the completion of a pretraining assessment allows for the identification of individual differences among students and a consequent tailoring of the skills curriculum to the special needs of each child.

Specification of Student Objectives

After identification of each student's skills and training needs through the baseline assessment, the competency-centered trainer specifies individualized training objectives. Based on these objectives, the trainer then begins to provide systematic training through didactic instruction when appropriate, modeling through simulated or actual demonstration of needed skills, review of self-directed manuals or brief written protocols, when available and applicable, and watching films when practicable. Training is focused on one skill component (i.e., one step of the task analysis) at a time in predetermined sequence.

Provision of Systematic Training

Simulation

Use of simulations typically involves anatomically correct dolls. Usage has been shown to be a viable tool for training young children in procedural skills related to self-administration of prescribed medical care routines (e.g., self-suctioning of a tracheal tube, self-catheterization of a bladder, self-injection). Incorporation of simulations provides increased training opportunities, because simulations are typically less effortful, less time-consuming, and less anxiety-provoking than are "live" applications. In addition, simulations can often be staged as "a game" that better motivates the child to participate in training. Significantly, simulation training avoids exposing the child to potentially dangerous or frightening events that may arise during actual applications (e.g., procedural mistakes and mishaps) before the child's competent skill acquisition. Finally, and perhaps most importantly, simulations enable the child to refine the youngster's self-administration technique without risking harmful consequences resulting from a serious error during actual trials.

Typically, completion of simulation training is based on a predetermined mastery criterion, predicated on the curriculum objectives and the nature and importance of the skills undergoing training. For example, with a procedure as crucial as correct self-suctioning, the mastery criterion may be exceptionally stringent, such as correct demonstration of 100% of critical component skills in the appropriate sequence, including at least 90% of those skills deemed to be less than critical, across at least two consecutive rehearsal simulations.

Training in Criterion Situation(s)

On repeated demonstrated mastery in simulated situations, with the child consistently exhibiting facile, satisfactory, and independent completion on the entire procedure, the youngster is encouraged to commence a highly similar training sequence focused on actual application. As with simulation training, actual training and remedial loops continue until the child exhibits mastery of the entire self-care routine during role playing self-administrations staged to require successful completion of each of the critical skills identified during curriculum development, as did the preceding simulations.

Completion of Skill Rehearsals

Once training has occurred, the child is often given multiple opportunities to first practice (rehearse) the target skill or management routines in simulated situations designed for the child to encounter key decision points requiring demonstration of recently described or demonstrated skills in the correct sequence. During such simulations, scripts are typically provided to the child and caregiver by the trainer to ensure that the simulation elicits practice of all critical skills. For instance, if the focus of the training module is the handling of emergencies, the script would detail the most pertinent emergency situations into the skill rehearsal.

Repeated Measurement of Student Performance in Simulated and Criterion (Actual) Situations

Simulations

Following attainment of the mastery criterion on each step of the task analysis, a **probe** (or assessment) is administered for previously trained and untrained skills to evaluate if the child has acquired a specific skill through independent demonstration. During each probe, the child is asked to exhibit how to suction the doll. Responses are scored as correct or incorrect, just as during training trials. However, unlike the training trials, no feedback or praise is provided to the child for performance during the probes. If the child does not demonstrate 100% correct responses for the trained skills, the youngster receives additional simulation training on target skills that were previously taught but performed inaccurately during the probe. This process is repeated until mastery is demonstrated.

Criterion Situation(s)

Typically, with competency-based training paradigms, a real-life demonstration probe is conducted following the mastery attainment on each simulation to assess for generalization of training effects to actual self-administration. For instance, the child is encouraged to do the youngster's best, is advised to stop whenever the child prefers, and is then asked to demonstrate suctioning of an actual tracheostomy. As a precaution, a nurse specialist is present during these actual demonstration probes to supervise the procedure. The nurse specialist is to interrupt any incorrect, potentially unsafe response, allowing the child to continue the procedure at the point of the next required response. As with training trials and simulation probes, responses are scored as correct, incorrect, or as not attempted. Again, no feedback or consequences are provided to the child based on self-performance.

Follow-up Probes

Once the child demonstrates mastery during two consecutive actual demonstration probes on all skill components, multiple follow-up checks are conducted in home (and possibly school) settings to assess maintenance as well as generalization of the trained procedural skills. Each follow-up check is conducted in the same way as during actual probes. Remedial training is provided, if need is indicated. In addition, when practicable, the child is asked to routinely self-monitor performance of each step of the procedure, determining if it was performed correctly and independently, or correctly but with assistance from someone else. The child is provided with self-addressed, stamped envelopes for return of the completed self-monitoring checklists each week until satisfactory performance, verified by follow-up assessments, is documented.

Provision of Remedial Training, as Indicated

Simulation

If the child fails to demonstrate mastery either during simulated or criterion situations, remedial training ensues. Often the trainer may need to step into the role of child during a simulation to provide additional instruction and modeling or to share performance-based feedback in response to a student error. Indeed, remedial training usually consists of additional instruction and demonstration, role-playing, and specific performance-based feedback. Training for a particular skill, skill domain, or task sequence continues until the predetermined mastery criterion is achieved. Opportunities to review and consolidate recently acquired skills are provided frequently as the student demonstrates proficiency with an entire skill domain.

Criterion (Actual) Situations

If a child fails to meet mastery criterion in an actual demonstration probe for the skill component(s) trained, the youngster receives additional training. As with remedial simulation training, remedial real-life training consists of additional instructions and modeling, followed by rehearsal by the child while the trainer provides praise and corrective feedback. Training continues until the child demonstrates 100% correct responses in the target skill area(s) during actual demonstration probes. Thereafter, simulation training followed by the role play training is initiated for the next step of the task analysis.

MOTIVATIONAL SYSTEMS

Self-care can be challenging for even the most highly motivated child. In many cases, a child initially balks at the prospect of self-administering a recommended care routine. The child's reluctance to self-administer may be related to fear and anxiety, to the child's opposition to or defiance of authority, or simply to the youngster's history of being able to rely on adults for care. The child may lack confidence, or may be aware that any newly found proficiency may lead to other changes, such as a change in school placement or the loss of a valued aide or nurse.

When the child fails to take the recommended initiative or becomes noncooperative, it is often necessary to design individually tailored motivational systems. These systems typically provide positive reinforcement by offering the child access to preferred objects, events, activities, or treats contingent on the youngster's cooperative effort and/or skill demonstration in actual practice. On occasion, motivational techniques also include the temporary withdrawal of privileges (e.g., the opportunity to visit the hospital's video arcade) or brief time-outs if the child refuses to complete an indicated procedure. However, optimal motivational systems do not typically include admonishment, lectures, yelling, reprimanding, bribing, ("cutting deals"), "talking things through," or spanking.

If a child has difficulty in managing self-care, it usually is necessary to arrange the circumstances surrounding the opportunity for the child to self-administer into an ultimatum. For instance, the child is informed that there is a deadline for the youngster to self-administer the target procedure. If the youngster does not meet the announced deadline, the child forfeits a certain privilege, and the staff (e.g., caregivers, visiting nurses, shift nurses, etc.) proceeds to administer the procedures themselves. Under these conditions, the majority of children not only promise to self-administer—they actually do! And, when they do, the adult care providers lavish the child with numerous acknowledgments, acts of approval, and special privileges. Typically, once the child breaks through and self-administers the procedure three to five times in succession without difficulty or challenging behavior, the child continues to self-administer satisfactorily, with only occasional coaching or discipline required thereafter.

EVALUATING OUTCOMES OF COMPETENCY-BASED CURRICULA

The construction and conduct of a training curriculum are but two of the critical components of an effective educational program. Another essential ingredient is a valid, reliable evaluation component. Comparison of pre- and post-training data enables trainers to determine whether students have acquired targeted skills. Problems can and often do arise if youngsters are said to be trained when data are not available to substantiate that they have, in fact, learned those skills purportedly developed through the training program. Attendance at or participation in a curriculum also does not ensure that the requisite skills have been learned. Even passing oral or written quizzes, or role plays (e.g., simulations alone), does not guarantee that skill acquisition has occurred. Only through direct evaluation of student performance can a skills training program be judged to be effective. Hence, one of the defining characteristics of a competency-based training paradigm is that student performance is assessed repeatedly in criterion (actual) as well as simulated situations, before, during, and after training.

EFFICIENCY OF COMPETENCY-BASED TRAINING

Many persons unfamiliar with competency-based curricula incorrectly assume that such curricula are necessarily time- and labor-intensive and, consequently, are impractical. Granted, the development of these curricula is often slow and methodical, thereby increasing the expense of the design and construction of the prototype. However, because competency-based curricula are exceptionally well-defined operationally and are optimally designed to be systematic and thorough, as well as skills-focused, the curricula are typically shown to be efficient as well as effective. In other words, the ultimate cost-effectiveness of a competency-based curriculum is demonstrated rapidly as it is disseminated to, adopted by, and replicated with multiple trainers and students. Indeed, if skill acquisition is the goal of (re)habilitation, then competency-based curricula are clearly among the most cost-beneficial, given that many other curricula never achieve the desired outcome (i.e., skills procurement) in the first place.

SOCIAL VALIDATION OF COMPETENCY-BASED CURRICULA

The comprehensive evaluation of a competency-based training model routinely includes a social validation. Typically, a consumer satisfaction questionnaire is administered not only to the child, but also to the trainers (e.g., caregivers, teachers, nurses, and other professionals). Frequently, respondents are asked to rate their degree of satisfaction with the training curriculum on multiple items, such as questions about the quality and amount of training, the extent to which independent mastery was achieved, the impact of training upon the student's self-esteem, whether or not the student would recommend the curriculum to other students, and so on.

CASE STUDY

Rather than considering Lisa and Frank (introduced in Chapter 1), whose developmental status prior to decannulation was not sufficient to perform the tasks described below, the key features of a competency-based curriculum will be illustrated through a description of a recently validated curriculum designed to teach children with tracheostomies to suction their tracheal tubes (Derrickson, Neef, & Parrish, 1991).

Based on anecdotal assertions in the previous medical and nursing literature that perhaps some children with tracheotomies could learn to self-administer their tracheostomy care routines, Derrickson and colleagues were intrigued with the prospect that a competency-based curriculum may be sufficient for independent skill acquisition by young children in selected cases. In the context of conducting a preliminary investigation employing an intrasubject experimental design (a multiple baseline design across both participants and skill domains), Derrickson et al. (1991) enrolled two boys and two girls between the ages of 5 and 8 years. Each had undergone tracheostomy during infancy. Primary medical diagnoses included Klippel-Feil Syndrome, bilateral vocal cord paralysis, **subglottic and/or tracheal stenosis**, and **tracheomalacia.** Two of the children had failed to respond acceptably to removal of the tracheostomy.

Each of the children demonstrated fine motor skills at the developmental age of 4 years or older, with collateral cognitive abilities ranging from 4 to beyond 5 years. Two of the children attended typical classrooms; the other two were enrolled in preschools for children with developmental disabilities. Two of the children had private nurses; the other two were managed exclusively by family or school personnel.

Baseline

Before beginning their curriculum, Derrickson et al. (1991) gave each of the four children enrolled in their study multiple opportunities to demonstrate their skills in suctioning, both with an anatomically correct doll and actual demonstrations with themselves. Mean percentage correct responses across each of the identified skill areas during baseline for probes with the doll ranged from 7.5% to 58.7%, with observed actual performance competence ranging from 8.1% to 53.5%. Hence, Derrickson and her colleagues documented that each child required training to achieve mastery and that children were most likely to demonstrate skills of gathering

and assembling equipment and cleaning up to a greater extent than
the suctioning procedure, per se.

Training

Derrickson et al.'s (1991) peer-reviewed task analysis yielded
three or four targeted skills domains for each enrolled child (Table
12-2). The first component, gathering and assembling equipment,
consisted of getting needed materials, washing hands, pouring water
in a cup, attaching the catheter to the suction machine, and putting
on a glove. The second component, administering oxygen and
normal saline solution, consisted of administering oxygen to the
tracheostomy via an ambu bag for three breaths and administering
three drops of normal saline solution to the tracheostomy before
suctioning. The third component, intermittent suctioning, entailed
inserting a catheter into the tracheostomy to a premarked length
without suctioning, applying intermittent suctioning while slowly
withdrawing the catheter in a rotating motion, readministering
oxygen between suctioning, and cleaning the catheter with water
between successive uses. The fourth skill component, cleaning up,
involved discarding nonreusable equipment, putting the catheter,
glove, and cup into the waste can, appropriately storing durable
equipment, and washing hands.

TABLE 12-2. Task analysis of self-suctioning skills.

SKILL	CORRECT RESPONSES
1. Gathering and assembling equipment	1.1 Child gets materials. 1.2 Child washes hands. 1.3 Child pours water in cup. 1.4 Child attaches catheter to machine. 1.5 Child puts on glove (sterile technique).
2. Administering oxygen (O_2)	2.1 Child regulates flow of oxygen (5-7/ml). Caregiver adminsters 3 breaths of O_2. Uses ambu bag, if needed. 2.2 Child administers drops of normal saline solution.
3. Intermittent suctioning	3.1 Child turns on suction machine (80-120 mm). 3.2 Child inserts catheter into tracheostomy at premarked length w/o suctioning. 3.3 Child applies intermittent suctioning, withdrawing catheter using rotation. 3.4 Child readministers oxygen, if needed. 3.5 Child cleans catheter in water.
4. Discarding equipment	4.1 Child puts disposable materials in waste can. 4.2 Child washes hands. 4.3 Child puts equipment away.

At the onset of training, the children were told that they could learn to suction their tracheostomies and were informed that each would first "help the doll to suction." Simulation training ensued, one step of the task analysis at a time. Training sessions were conducted individually, with the necessary materials at hand. The child was first informed of the step that the youngster needed to perform (e.g., "First, you put this tube in the doll's neck without sucking anything out."). The trainer then modeled the completion of the step using the doll, while verbalizing the actions being taken (e.g., "Watch me while I put the tube in the doll's neck without suctioning").

A learning (or performance) trial was initiated by restoring all needed materials to the initial location and condition. The child was then requested to suction the doll's tracheostomy and to tell what was being done to the doll. The doll was handled from a sitting position on the child's lap, with the doll facing away from the child to simulate the angles for the performance of actual self-suctioning. None of the children used a mirror to facilitate their viewing of the procedures. The duration of each trial ranged from 10 to 20 minutes.

A correct response by the child was followed immediately by descriptive praise (e.g., "That's it! You found the hole and put the tube in!"). Subsequent to an incorrect response, the trainer provided helpful feedback and again demonstrated the correct response with the doll. Next, a remedial trial on the step performed incorrectly was completed. This sequence continued until the child completed the step independently and correctly. Then, the next step for the skill area targeted for training was presented.

Procedural adaptations were made on an individualized basis, being tailored to the specific needs of each child. For example, a visual cue (i.e., stamp or star) was applied on the dominant hand of three of the children to assist them in selecting the correct hand for holding the catheter. With these same children, the trainer also tapped the child's thumb that was to administer suction as a reminder to the child to keep the thumb off the suction port during the insertion of the catheter into the tracheostomy.

Repeated Measurement of Student Performance

Subsequent to training related to each skill domain, Derrickson et al. (1991) conducted assessments of the child's performance of both trained and untrained procedural steps on the doll. During each probe using the doll, the child was asked to demonstrate how to suction. No performance-based feedback or differential conse- quences were provided, other than to thank the child for participating at the end of the probe. If the child did not exhibit mastery of all previously trained steps, then the youngster received additional simulation training for steps performed incorrectly. This remedial process was repeated until mastery of all trained steps was achieved.

Motivational System

As a motivational tool, Derrickson et al. (1991) instituted a star chart system for each child, to acknowledge the child's participation in the training curriculum. At the conclusion of each training session, whether it be a simulation or an actual application, the child was given a star if the youngster had been cooperative while helping the doll or doing the demonstration. At the end of each week, if the child had earned a star during every session, the youngster was permitted to select a special sticker.

Evaluation of Outcome

Derrickson et al. (1991) employed an intrasubject time-series design to determine if the enrolled children had acquired the target skills and continued to correctly practice them in home and school settings following the completion of the training sequence. The researchers' analyses revealed that the performance of each child improved immediately following training in each successive skill area. Each child achieved the 100% mastery criterion in all skill domains. Furthermore, generalization of the effects of simulated training with the doll to actual self-suctioning was also observed in all skill components for all children. Performance gains were documented in home and school settings, with no remedial training required with any of the children during follow-up, which ranged in duration from 2 to 6 weeks. In fact, for all children, mean percentage correct responses across all skills ranged from 92% to 100% during follow-up.

Evaluation of Efficiency

Derrickson et al. (1991) included an analysis of the number and duration of training sessions necessary to reach mastery criterion in their assessment of the efficacy of their competency-based paradigm. Their analyses revealed that the mean number of sessions needed to reach criterion was 8.0 (range, 2 to 24) for the gathering and assembling of equipment, 16.5 (range, 5 to 30) for the application of suctioning, and 2.8 (range, 2 to 4) for clean-up. Conservative estimates of total training time, based on the number and duration

264 THE CARE OF CHILDREN WITH LONG-TERM TRACHEOSTOMIES

of training sessions ranged from 1 hour, 30 minutes to 18 hours, 40 minutes.

Social Validation

Derrickson et al. (1991) sent consumer satisfaction questionnaires to the caregivers, teachers, and nurses who observed the training sessions with the participating children. The opinions expressed by these respondents suggested that the adult care providers were quite pleased with the quality and amount of training the children received, as well as with perceived increases in the children's self-esteem. More importantly, each of the participating children indicated enjoying learning to suction and, as a result of training, they could help their caregiver with the suctioning procedure. Each stated that other children with tracheostomies should learn to suction themselves.

CONCLUSIONS

Competency-based training programs routinely meet the most important standards against which any curriculum can be judged: Comprehensive, experimentally validated (i.e., data-based and data-driven), cost-effective, and exportable. It is through the systematic construction, validation, implementation, and evaluation of such programs that professionals will gradually but inexorably enable citizens who are technologically assisted, including those with long-term tracheostomies, to acquire those skills necessary to achieve optimal independent function.

ACKNOWLEDGMENTS

This work was partially supported by NICHHD Mental Retardation Research Center Core Grant No. P30 DH26979, MCH Grant No. MCJ 9124, and MCH Grant No. MCJ 429308. The positions expressed in this work are solely those of the author and are not intended to represent any endorsement by a federal funding agency.

REFERENCES

Babbitt, R., Parrish, J., Brierley, P., & Kohr, M. (1991). Teaching developmentally disabled children with chronic illness to swallow prescribed capsules. *Journal of Developmental and Behavioral Pediatrics, 12(4)*, 229-235.

Bosch, J.D., & Cuyler, J.P. (1987). Home care of the pediatric tracheostomy: Our experience. *Journal of Otolaryngology, 16,* 120-122.

Calkins, C., Gibson, B., Grosko, J., & Bueker, J. (1982). *Respite care adapted for deaf-blind population: Training manual.* Kansas City, University of Missouri-Kansas City Institute, university affiliated facility.

Derrickson, J., Neef, N.A., & Parrish, J.M. (1991). Teaching self-administration of suctioning to children with tracheostomies. *Journal of Applied Behavior Analysis, 24,* 563-570.

Feldman, W.S., Manella, K.J., & Varni, J.W. (1983). A behavioral parent training program for single mothers of physically handicapped children. *Child Care, Health, & Development, 9,* 157-168.

Friedman, M.M. (1986). *Family nursing: Theory and assessment* (2nd ed.) Norwalk, CN: Appleton-Century-Crofts.

Gage, M.A., Fredericks, H.D., Johnson-Dorn, N., & Lindley-Southard, B. (1982). Inservice training for staff of group homes and work activity centers serving developmentally disabled adults. *Journal of the Association for the Severely Handicapped, 7,* 60-70.

Gross, A.M., Eudy, C., & Drabman, R.S. (1982). Training parents to be physical therapists with their physically handicapped child. *Journal of Behavioral Medicine, 5,* 321-327.

Jenkins, S., Stephens, B., & Sternberg, L. (1980). The use of parents as parent trainees of handicapped children. *Education and Training of the Mentally Retarded, 15,* 256-263.

Jennings, P. (1988). Nursing and home aspects of the care of a child with a tracheostomy. *Journal of Laryngology and Otology,* (Suppl. 17), 25-29.

Kennedy, A.H., Johnson, W.G., & Sturdevant, E.W. (1982). An educational program for families of children with tracheostomies. *Maternal Child Health Nursing Journal, 7(1),* 42-49.

Kennelly, C. (1990). Tracheostomy care: Parents as learners. *Maternal and Child Nursing, 12,* 264-267.

Kohrman, A.F. (in press). Psychological issues in pediatric home care. In M.J. Mehlman & S.J. Younger (Eds.) *Issues in high technology home care: A guide for decision making* (pp. 1-35). Baltimore: National Health Publishing.

Lichtenstein, M.A. (1986). Pediatric home tracheostomy care: A parent's guide. *Pediatric Nursing, 12(1),* 41-48, 69.

Lukenbill, R., Lillie, B., Sanddal, N., Hulme, J., Calkins, C., & McKibben, M. (1976). *Respite care training manual.* Helena, Developmental Disabilities Training Institute.

Macy, D.J., Solomon, G.S., Schoen, M., & Galey, G.S. (1983). The DEBT Project: Early intervention for handicapped children and their parents. *Exceptional Children,* 447-448.

Neef, N.A., Parrish, J.M., Egel, A.L., & Sloan, M.E. (1986). Training respite care providers for families with handicapped children: An experimental analysis and validation of an instructional package. *Journal of Applied Behavior Analysis, 6,* 131-166.

Neef, N.A., Parrish, J.M., Hannigan, K.F., Page, T.J., & Iwata, B.A. (1986). Teaching self-catheterization skills to children with neurogenic bladder complications. *Journal of Applied Behavior Analysis, 22,* 237-243.

O'Dell, S.L., Blackwell, L.J., Larcen, S.W., & Hogan, J.L. (1977). Competency-based training for severely behaviorally handicapped children and their parents. *Journal of Autism and Childhood Schizophrenia, 7,* 231-242.

Parrish, J.M., Egel, A.L., & Neef, N.A. (1986). Respite care provider training: A competency-based approach. In C. Salisbury (Ed.), *Respite care provider training: Current practices and directions for research* (pp. 117-142). Baltimore: Paul H. Brookes.

Richman, G.S., Ponticas, Y., Page, T.J., & Epps, S. (1986). Simulation procedures for teaching independent menstrual care to mentally retarded persons. *Applied Research in Mental Retardation, 7,* 21-35.

Rickert, V., Sottolano, D., Parrish, J., Riley, A., Hunt, F., & Pelco, L. (1988). Training parents to become better behavior managers: The need for a competency-based approach. *Behavior Modification, 12(4),* 475-496.

Riley, A.W., Parrish, J.M., & Cataldo, M.F. (1989). Training parents to meet the needs of children with medical or physical handicaps. In C.E. Schaefer & J.M. Briesmeister (Eds.), *Handbook of parent training: Parents as co-therapists for children's behavior problems* (pp. 305-336). New York: Wiley.

Ruben, R.J., Newton, L., Jornsay, D., Stein, R., Chambers, H., Liquori, J., & Lawrence, C. (1982). Home care of the pediatric patient with a tracheostomy. *Annals of Otology, Rhinology, and Laryngology, 91,* 633-640.

Salzinger, K., Feldman, R., & Portnoy, S. (1970). Training parents of brain-injured children in the use of operant conditioning procedures. *Behavior Therapy, 1,* 4-32.

Sandler, A., Coren, A., & Thurman, S.K. (1983). A training program for parents of handicapped preschool children: Effects upon mother, father, and child. *Exceptional Children,* 355-358.

Schreiner, M.S., Donar, M.E., & Kettrick, R.G. (1987). Pediatric home mechanical ventilation. *Pediatric Clinics of North America, 34,* 47-60.

Singer, G.H.S., & Irvin, L.K. (Ed.) (1989). *Support for caregiving families: Enabling positive adaptation to disability.* Baltimore: Paul H. Brookes.

Singer, L.T., Wood, R., & Lambert, S. (1985). Developmental follow-up of long-term infant tracheostomy: A preliminary report. *Journal of Developmental and Behavioral Pediatrics, 6(3),* 132-136.

Stool, S.E., & Beebe, J.K. (1973). Tracheostomy in infants and children. *Current Problems in Pediatrics, 3,* 3-33.

Tatro v. State of Texas, 104 S. Ct. 3371 (1984).

Watson, L., & Uzzell, R. (1980). A program for teaching behavior modification skills to institutional staff. *Applied Research in Mental Retardation, 1,* 41-53.

Weitz, S.E. (1981). A code for assessing teaching skills of parents of developmentally disabled children. *Journal of Autism and Developmental Disorders, 12(1),* 13-24.

Ziarnik, J.P., & Bernstein, G. (1982). A critical examination of the effect of inservice training on staff performance. *Mental Retardation, 20,* 109-114.

Zlomke, L., & Benjamin, V. (1983). Staff inservice: Measuring effectiveness through client behavior change. *Education and Training of the Mentally Retarded, 18,* 125-130.

SECTION V

SUMMARY

13

A Circle of Care

Ken M. Bleile, Cynthia Solot, Laura Fus, and Shari A. Miller

INTRODUCTION

In the last 10 to 15 years advances in medical care have created the possibility of sustaining life in critically ill neonates and infants with the aid of **tracheostomy** and ventilator support. In extending the boundaries of medicine, society has created a new population of children with special needs whose lives are dependent on the machinery that breathes for them as well as on the care of the professionals to whom their lives and development are entrusted.

The chapters in this book described the provision of care to children with **long-term tracheostomies** and those who receive **ventilation assistance.** This chapter is an overview of this care and indicates the parts of the book in which the major aspects of care are discussed. The following topics are addressed:

- Areas of care
- Qualifications of health care providers
- Phases in care

AREAS OF CARE

Care is provided to children with long-term tracheostomies in hope of improving their quality of life. Physical health is a prerequisite to a good quality of life, but not sufficient for a life that most people would find enjoyable. Therefore, the health care team strives to also improve the child's life in the developmentally critical areas of communication, movement, socialization, cognition, feeding, behavior, and self-help. Table 13-1 lists the chapters in which pertinent therapeutic goals are covered. In all tables in this chapter, the chapters most directly pertinent to a topic are in bold face.

QUALIFICATIONS OF HEALTH CARE PROVIDERS

Because the physical and developmental needs of children with long-term tracheostomies are too complex to be managed by any single discipline, care is typically provided by a team consisting of the child's caregivers and representatives from such different professions as medicine, nursing, education, speech-language pathology, and occupational and physical therapy. Some teams are sometimes also fortunate to include representatives from recreational therapy and nutrition.

In addition to having excellent qualifications in their area of expertise, all health care providers best provide safe and integrated care by having knowledge of several more general topics, including the range of developmental outcomes of children with long-term tracheostomies, ethical issues likely to arise in the provision of care, health care precautions that need to be in place when providing care, the children's rights to education services, and the criteria and goals that must be met as the child advances from the acute care setting to the community. Table 13-2 lists the chapters in which these topics are discussed.

TABLE 13-1. Areas of Care.

CRITERIA	PERTINENT CHAPTERS
Physical Care	Chapters **2**, **3**, & **11**
Communication	Chapters 2, 3, 4, & **6**
Movement	Chapters **4** & 8
Cognition	Chapters 6, **7**, & 8
Feeding	Chapter 5
Behavior	Chapters **7** & **12**
Socialization	Chapters 6, **7**, 8, & 10
Self-Help	Chapters 3, 5, 6, 7, 8, 10, & **12**

TABLE 13-2.   Areas of Knowledge beyond Professional expertise.

CRITERIA	PERTINENT CHAPTERS
Population characteristics	Chapter 1
Developmental outcome	Chapter 1
Ethical issues	Chapter 1
Health care precautions	Chapters 2, 3, & **4**
Rights to education	Chapter 9
Hospital and community requirements	Chapter 13

PHASES IN CARE

The health care team forms what is described in the management of HIV/AIDS patients as a Circle of Care around the child. Early in the child's hospital admission, the primary goal of care is to maintain the child's physical well-being and, when possible, to provide emotional and practical assistance for the child's caregivers. Developmental interventions are provided only as the child's medical condition improves.

The child enters the (re)habilitation phase of care when the youngster is medically stable and the tracheostomy is stable and mature, as evidenced by a successful first tracheostomy change after placement. The most typical goals of admission to a rehabilitation unit are to train caregivers in tracheostomy care, provide intensive therapy, and to help meet the child's nutritional needs. Table 13-3 lists the chapters in which these issues are addressed.

In all but the rarest situations, children with long-term tracheostomies benefit most from being home with their families. Therefore, children are often placed in the community with their

TABLE 13-3.   Sample goals while in a rehabilitation setting.

GOALS	PERTINENT CHAPTERS
Training of caregivers in tracheostomy care and overall physical care of the child	Chapters **11** & **12**
An intense period of rehabilitation directed at anticipated difficulties associated with tracheostomy	Chapters **4, 5, 6, 7,** & **8**
Nutritional rehabilitation of the child with pre-existing growth failure possible from longstanding airway obstruction	Chapter 5

tracheostomy still in place. Preparing a family to provide care in the home to a child with a long-term tracheostomy is one of the most difficult aspects of care provision. Table 13-4 lists the goals that must be met in preparing a child for discharge and the chapters most pertinent to attainment of these goals.

While the management of the tracheostomy remains critical after the child returns to the community, the focus of care shifts to education as the child's medical problems recede. The criteria that must be met to maintain a child in the community are listed in Table 13-5, along with the chapters that are most pertinent to these topics.

CONCLUSIONS

Children with long-term tracheostomies often have complex medical and developmental needs, and, for this reason, their care is typically managed by a team of health care providers. Along with the child's caregivers, this team forms a Circle of Care around the child.

TABLE 13-4. Sample preparations to be completed prior to discharge from a rehabilitation setting to the community.

PREPARATION	PERTINENT CHAPTERS
Caregiver has demonstrated the ability to success-fully care for the child at home	Chapters **10, 11,** & **12**
Caregiver has repeatedly demonstrated the ability to successfully carry out specific care procedures, and to react appropriately in simulated crisis situations	Chapters **11 & 12**
Home adaptions have been made, and child's home equipment is in place	Chapters 8, **10,** & 11
Adaptive equipment is appropriate and functional	Chapters 4, **6,** & **10**
Educational arrangements or early intervention servi-ces have been made	Chapters **4, 5, 6, 7, 8,** & **9**
Home health care has been arranged	Chapters **10** & 11
Home instructions have been written and given to family, nursing agency, supplier of respiratory equipment, and community therapists	Chapters **4, 5, 6, 7, 8, 10, 11, & 12**
The family demonstrates an understanding of the medical follow-up required, and the responsibili-ties of the individuals and organizations that will be providing services in the home	Chapters **10, 11,** & **12**
Funding is available and adequate for home care	Chapter **10**

TABLE 13-5.   Sample criteria needed to maintain a child with an in-place tracheostomy in the community.

CRITERIA	PERTINENT CHAPTERS
The child is medically stable, has a stable airway, and the level of respiratory support provides sufficient reserve to allow participation in activities of daily living and developmental advancement	Chapters **2, 3, 10,** & 11
The child's nutritional regimen promotes normal to accelerated growth	Chapter 5
The caregivers understand their child's diagnosis and prognosis	Chapter **1** & **10**
The child is receiving early intervention or educational services	Chapters **4, 5, 6, 7, 8,** & **9**
The family is willing and capable of meeting their child's special needs	Chapters **10**, 11, & 12
There is financial support available to fund equipment, supplies, and home care personnel	Chapter 11

GLOSSARY

Glossary of Frequently Encountered Technical Terminology

Laura Fus

Acute respiratory failure: Sudden inability to provide adequate gas exchange during respiration; demands support of ventilation to sustain life

Air hunger: Gasping for air

Alternative communication system: System used in place of vocalizations

Anoxia: Condition in which body tissues receive inadequate oxygen amounts

Arterial oxygen saturation: Amount of oxygen in arterial blood supply

Asphyxia: Suffocation; oxygen prevented from reaching tissues by obstruction of or damage to any part of the respiratory system

Aspirated: Withdrawal of fluid from body by suctioning

Aspiration: The inhalation of foreign material (typically, food or liquid) into the lungs

Atelectasis: Collapse of lung alveoli

Automatic phasic bite-release response: Oral reflex pattern elicited when tactile stimulation is provided to the molar surface

Barotrauma: Injury resulting from repeated application of positive pressure on the airways through young and damaged airways

Baseline: Level of skills before implementation of treatment

Bronchopulmonary dysplasia (BPD): Chronic lung disease of prematurity resulting from premature lungs, the trauma of ventilation, and the toxicity of supplemental oxygen

275

Bronchoscope: Instrument used to look into the trachea and bronchi

Bronchoscopy: Visual examination of trachea and bronchus

Buccal speech: Using air trapped in the cheeks to produce a source of vibration

Cannula: Tube

Cannula occlusion: Closing off the stoma temporarily with the finger to facilitate voicing

Cardiac anomaly: Disorder of, relating to, or affecting the heart

Cardiac failure: Cessation of effective pumping action of the heart

Cardiomegaly: Enlargement of the heart, usually in response to a need to increase pressures to pump blood into the lungs or to the rest of the body

Carina: Bifurcation of trachea into right and left bronchi

Case manager: Coordinator of evaluations and assessments; also support and strengthen family functioning, including linking them up with community support

Chronic mechanical ventilation (CMV): Use of a ventilator, usually for more than one month, with the expectation that it will be needed for at least several months or for 28 days or more

Chronic respiratory failure: Inability to eliminate carbon dioxide and, usually, to sustain adequate oxygen levels

Classic conditioning theory: A previously learned neutral stimulus becomes a conditioned stimulus when presented with an unconditioned stimulus

Competency-based training paradigms: Acquisition and maintenance of specific skills through performance of skills as learning occurs

Concentration: Amount of oxygen delivered

Conductive hearing loss: Hearing impairment due to failure of sound pressure waves to reach the cochlea through normal air conduction channels

Congenital anomalies: Disorder present at birth, whether inherited or caused by an environmental factor

Congenital hypoventilation syndrome: Syndrome in which a child is born breathing abnormally slow, resulting in increased blood carbon dioxide

Continuous flow ventilators: Steady air supply at the patient's airway

Continuous positive airway pressure (CPAP): Machine or other device that maintains a constant pressure throughout the airway, preventing collapse of the lung by easing the work of breathing in and out

Contractures: Fibrosis of muscle tissue producing shrinkage and shortening of muscle, with loss of strength

Craniofacial anomalies: Malformation affecting both the cranium and face

Chronic mechanical ventilation (CMV): See long-term (chronic) mechanical ventilation

Croup: Inflammation and obstruction of the larynx in children younger than 2 years, usually a result of viral respiratory tract infection

Cyanosis: Bluish discoloration of skin and mucous membranes resulting from inadequate amounts of oxygen in the blood

Decannulation: Removal of tracheostomy tube

Diaphragm: Muscular and tendonous partition separating the thoracic and abdominal cavities

Doliocephaly: Flattened, narrow, elongated head shape

Down-size: The process of using progressively smaller tracheostomy tubes in a patient prior to decannulation

Down syndrome: Mental subnormality due to chromosome defect

Dysphagia: Difficulty in swallowing

Early intervention play: Structured daily program of activities in an interdisciplinary environment facilitating development of communication and functional skills

Education for All Handicapped Children Act (PL 99-142): Provision of free appropriate education to all children with handicaps, 3-21 years old, including evaluation and assessment, right to due process of law, and financial support for educational services

Education of Handicapped Act Amendments (PL 99-457): Amendments encouraging the development and implementation of early intervention services for children birth to 3 years old and their families

Electrolarynx: Electronic device designed to produce a vibratory sound source which can be transmitted into the vocal tract

Encephalopathy: Any disease of the brain

Endotracheal tube: Plastic tube inserted through the mouth and into the larynx to provide ventilation to the lungs and to help aspirate secretions

Endotracheal intubation: Placement of a plastic tube through the mouth and the larynx

Endoscopy: Visual examination of airway

Epiglottitis: Inflammation of mucous membrane of epiglottis, which may obstruct the airflow to the lungs

Epithelialized: Formation of tissue lining hollow structures (i.e., stoma)

Esophageal speech: Speech produced by swallowing air and then releasing it into the throat again

Esophageal stage: Third stage of swallowing, in which the bolus is moved down the esophagus to the gastrointestinal tract

Fenestrated cannula: Tracheostomy tube with a hole (fenestra) at the top of the bend of the tube to allow vocalization

Full-scale IQ: Intelligence quotient based on verbal skills and motor/performance skills

Gastroesophageal reflux (GER): Backward flow of stomach contents into the esophagus

Gastrostomy tube: Feeding tube inserted directly into the stomach via surgical incision through the abdomen

Granulation tissue: Mass that forms as part of the body's inflammatory response to a foreign body

Head trauma: Injury to the head may require tracheostomy placement due to the needs of hyperoxygenation immediately following the accident or for lung collapse as the result of the accident

Humidivent: Filter attached to the exterior end of the tracheal tube that collects the patient's expired moisture to humidify inspired air when the child is not attached to a ventilator set-up

Hyaline membrane disease: Surfactant-deficiency disease of premature infants

Hydrocephalus: Abnormal increase in amount of cerebrospinal fluid within brain ventricles

Hypertrophic scarring: Enlarged scar formation

Hypotonia: Lack of muscle tone

Individualized Education Plan (IEP): Written statement for a child who is handicapped, describing educational objectives for the child and special services to be provided

Individualized Family Service Plan (IFSP): Plan developed by caregivers and family to outline specifics of services for children with handicaps and their families

Inflated cuff tracheal tube: Tracheal tube with air bladder at the end of the tube that can be inflated to different pressures to seal a leak

Interdisciplinary: Groups of professionals who independently perform tasks or services, yet communicate to coordinate efforts

Intermittent flow ventilators: Ventilators requiring patient effort to draw air through an intake hose

Intraventricular hemorrhage: Bleeding within the brain ventricles

Jejunostomy tube: Tube surgically inserted through the abdomen into the jejunum (part of small intestine)

Keloid: Hypertrophic (thick) scar

Laryngeal diversion: Surgical procedure in which trachea is divided and the lower segment is sutured to neck skin to form a permanent tracheostoma

Laryngeal neoplasm: Laryngeal growth or tumor

Laryngomalacia: Condition of airway obstruction secondary to floppy and/or redundant tissue overlying the laryngeal opening

Laryngotracheoplasty: Surgical procedure in which airway is opened and cartilage graft is placed to augment tracheal lumen

Long-term (chronic) mechanical ventilation (CMV): Equipment required to maintain a flow of air into and out of lungs for a minimum of 28 days

Long-term tracheostomy: Presence of a tracheostomy for 28 days or longer

Manual communication: Sign language

Mechanical ventilation: See: long-term mechanical ventilation

Methylene blue screening: Special assessment for aspiration, with methylene blue dye added to food, and secretions from suctioning are examined for traces of dye following feeds

Mode: How the ventilator operates with respect to patient effort

Mucus plug: Obstruction of airway by thick mucus

Multidisciplinary: Groups of professionals performing related tasks but working independent of each other

Myelomeningocele: Neural tube defect in which the spinal cord and nerve roots are exposed, resulting in constant risk of infection, paralysis and numbness of the legs, and urinary incontinence

Nasogastric tube: Feeding tube inserted through the nose into the stomach

Negative pressure ventilator: Machine that assists respiration by exerting a sucking motion on the outside of the chest, allowing the lungs to fill with air

Negative reinforcement: Removing something aversive

Neurological sequelae: Disorder of nervous system resulting from preceding disease or accident

Neuromuscular disorder: Condition resulting from the lack of synapse between a motor neuron and the muscle fiber which inhibits the triggering of muscle action

Nonverbal intelligence: Aspects of intelligence that are not language based (i.e., perceptual-motor)

NPO: Medical abbreviation for not per oral (not by mouth)

Occupational therapy: Fine motor development, cognitive and perceptual maturation, and psychosocial adjustment for developing functional skills for play, self-care, and school

Operant conditioning theory: Method of changing behavior in which the experimenter waits for the response to be conditioned to occur spontaneously, immediately after which the subject is reinforced

Oral stage: First stage of swallowing in which the mouth is oriented to the bolus

Peak Inspiratory Pressure: See PIP

PEEP (Positive End Expiratory Pressure): Small pressure at end of expiration, often expressed as PIP/PEEP

Percussion and postural drainage (P&PD): Procedure of clapping on child's chest to loosen secretions so they can be coughed up or suctioned from tracheostomy tube

Perinatal: During the birth process

Pharyngeal stage: Second stage of swallowing, in which the bolus moves through the pharynx to the esophagus

Phonation assessment: Evaluation to determine if voicing is possible

Phrenic nerve: Nerve that supplies muscles of the diaphragm

Physical therapy: Focuses on gross motor skill, balance, and posture as it relates to the ability to mobilize in the environment

Pierre Robin syndrome: Craniofacial anomaly often associated with airway obstruction

PIP (Peak Inspiratory Pressure): Peak pressure during inspiration, often expressed as PIP/PEEP

Pneumothorax: Collapsed lung (free air in the chest cavity)

PO: Medical abbreviation for per oral (by mouth)

Positive End Expiratory Pressure: See PEEP

Positive pressure ventilator: Machine that forces air into the lungs through a tube in the nose, mouth, or throat

Positive reinforcement: Receiving something desirable

Prematurity: Birth of a baby before full-term, defined as one weighing less than 2,500 g

Pressure: Strength of ventilation

Pressure ventilators: Ventilators allowing the operator to set the pressure of air which is forced into the lungs

Probe: Assessment of skill acquisition with no feedback given

Public Law 94-142: See: Education for All Handicapped Children Act

Public Law 99-457: See: Education of Handicapped Act Amendment

Public Law 100-146: Developmental Disabilities Assistance Act Amendments of 1987

Public Law 101-236: Individuals with Disabilities Education Amendments of 1990

Pulmonary insufficiency: Inadequate functioning of the lungs

Pulmonary vascular hypertension: Increase in the pressure and hence the workload of the right ventricle, which pumps blood into the lungs; results from diseased lungs, which narrow the blood vessels

Pulse oximeter: Monitor that displays heart rate and oxygen saturation level

Quadriplegia: Paralysis affecting all four limbs

Rales: Abnormal respiratory sounds heard in lungs

Rate: Number of breaths per minute

Residential school: Setting in which handicapped children live in the special school

Respiratory assessment: Determining respiratory rate, check vital signs, listen for breath sounds, check work of breathing, report changes

Respiratory distress: Condition in which the lungs are imperfectly expanded so breathing is rapid, labored, and shallow

Respiratory failure: Inadequacy in exchange of oxygen and carbon dioxide during respiration

Rooting: Head turning reaction when the perioral region is stroked

Sensorineural hearing loss: Hearing impairment resulting from pathological condition either in inner ear or nerve pathway between inner ear and brain stem

Sign language: System of communication by means of hand gestures

Skills checklist: List of all skills that a home care learner needs to master to safely care for child

Speaking valve: Any valve placed on the end of a tracheostomy tube to facilitate speech production

Special class: Setting in which the child spends most of the day in a special education class within a regular school

Special day school: Setting in which children spend the entire school day in special schools

State model waiver program: Option for funding home care for the child with a tracheostomy and/or a ventilator if insurance has been exhausted or child is on Medicaid

Stoma: The opening in the neck into which the tracheostomy tube is inserted

Subglottic stenosis: Narrowing of airway below larynx

Sucking pads: Fatty tissue appearing during the first 1-1/2 months in utero providing postural stability for the infant when sucking

Supine positioning: Lying on the back

Surfactant: Secretion of the lungs which lines the alveoli and prevents their collapse when alveoli are inflated

Synchronized intermittent mandatory ventilation (SIMV): Ventilation system with mechanism to sense the patient's inspiratory effort and to coordinate the ventilator with the patient effort

Task analysis: Step-by-step description of skills in prescribed management routine, with each step an observable and measurable action

Teaching contract: Predischarge home care teaching plan with schedule agreed upon by staff and caregivers

Therapeutic recreation: Intervention providing children with opportunities for play, learning, self-expression, family involvement, and peer interactions

Torticollis: Turning movement of the head that becomes more persistent until the head eventually is continually held to one side

Tracheal collar: External band around the neck used to secure tracheal tube through strings attached to the external portions of the apparatus

Tracheal lumen: The space inside of the trachea

Tracheal stenosis: Narrowing of airway at trachea

Tracheobronchial toilet: The clearing of tracheal secretions

Tracheocutaneous fistula: Abnormal opening to the trachea through the skin

Tracheoesophageal anomalies: Defect of the tracheal and esophageal structures

Tracheomalacia: Airway obstruction related to collapse of softened tracheal cartilages

Tracheostomy: The artificial opening created between the trachea and the anterior neck

Tracheostomy tube tract: Connection between neck skin and tracheal lumen through which the tracheostomy tube passes

Transdisciplinary: Groups of professionals who perform tasks by sharing information and roles

Treacher Collins' syndrome: Craniofacial anomaly often associated with airway obstruction

Ventilator assistance: Mechanical assistance to breathe

Very low birthweight: Usually defined as less than 1,500 g

Videofluoroscopic swallowing function study: Assessment to examine oral and pharyngeal motility during feeding, using food mixed with barium; the food's path is traced via videofluoroscopic radiology

Volume ventilators: Ventilators that allow the operator to set the tidal volume

Web: Thin membrane between two structures

Wheezing: Whistling respiratory sound

APPENDIX

Addresses

Organizations and companies referred to in the book:

Chapter 5
(Oral Motor and Feeding
Disorders)
Therapy Skill Builders
P. O. Box 42050
Tucson, AZ 85733
(602) 323-7500
spoons

Northcoast Medical, Inc.
187 Stauffer Blvd.
San Jose, CA 95125-1042
spoons

Chapter 6
(Communication Disorders)
Passy and Passy, Inc.
4521 Campus Drive, Suite 273
Irvine, CA 92715
Passy-Muir speaking valve

American Pharmaseal Company
American Hospital Supply
Corporation
Valencia, CA 91355-8900
Airlife "T" Adaptor speaking valve

Communicative Medical, Inc.
P. O. Box 8241
Spokane, WA 99203-0241
(800) 944-6801
electrolarynx

Chapter 8 (Recreation)
VACC Camp
Ventilator Assisted Children's Center
Miami Children's Hospital
6125 S. W. 31st Street
Miami, FL 33155
(305) 662-8222
summer camp for children receiving
ventilator assistance

SKIP Camp, Inc.
11208 Minnetonka Mills Road
Minnetonka, MN 55108
(612) 935-5581
summer camp for children with medical conditions

Sesame Place Challenge for Variety
Club
Variety Club
The Warwick
17th St. at Locust
Philadelphia, PA 19103
(215) 735-0803
developed community programs for
children with medical involvement

Other Addresses of Interest:

Association for the Care of
Children's Health
7910 Woodmont Ave, Suite 300
Bethesda, MD 20814
free listing of publications con-
cerning children with special
needs

The National Self-Help Clearinghouse
25 W. 43rd St.
New York, NY 10036
refers people to support groups
nationwide

Index